MW00951882

Renal Diet

COOKBOOK FOR BEGINNERS

Kidney-Friendly Recipes with Low Phosphorus.
Easy and Nutritious Dishes for a Healthy Renal System.
Delicious Meals to Support Your Kidney Health and Wellness.
Includes Guide with 30-Day Meal Plan

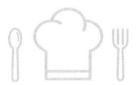

By EMILY KEMP

2023 Edition

Disclaimer

The book "RENAL DIET COOKBOOK FOR BEGINNERS" is meant to serve the readers with accurate and trustworthy data about the subject at hand. The buyer should understand that the publisher is not obligated to provide accounting, legal, or other specialized services concerning publishing. A qualified practitioner should be summoned if expert legal or professional guidance is required.

Every endeavor has been driven to ensure the accuracy of the information presented; nonetheless, the reader assumes all risk associated with the use or misuse of any policies, practices, or directives outlined herein, whether due to carelessness or otherwise. The author will not be held accountable in any way for any direct or indirect monetary or other losses incurred as a result of using the information included herein.

As of 2023, all rights to the eBook are held under copyright. Without the author's complete and signed written permission, information may not be copied, recorded, or transmitted electronically or mechanically.

Copyright© 2023 Emily Kemp

All right reserved.

Table of Contents

Chapter 11: MEAT RECIPES 103

Chapter 12: SOUPS 113

About author

EMILY KEMP is a registered dietitian and renal professional with more than ten years of experience helping patients manage kidney disease. She holds a degree in dietetics and completed her clinical training at a top hospital specializing in nephrology. Throughout her journey, Emily has experienced the impact of diet on kidney health. She is dedicated to assisting individuals with kidney disease to improve their diet and lifestyle through positive changes. She is enthusiastic about creating delicious and nutritious meals low in potassium, sodium, and phosphorus – essential nutrients that must carefully manage for people with kidney disease.

Emily has collaborated with many patients to develop personalized meal plans that fit their unique nutritional needs. Emily's healthy and easy-to-prepare recipes enable people with kidney disease to relish delicious and gratifying meals.

As an author, she is also committed to sharing her expertise with a broader audience. Her latest book, "Renal Diet Cookbook for Beginners," is a comprehensive guide. This cookbook is a vital resource for anyone who wants to enhance their kidney health through diet. It also includes a 30-day meal plan and uses affordable and accessible ingredients.

Introduction

Your kidneys are the unsung heroes of your body, silently working to keep you healthy and thriving

Kidney disease is a common and severe health condition affecting millions worldwide. The kidneys are crucial in filtering waste products from the blood, regulating electrolyte levels, and producing hormones that regulate blood pressure and red blood cell production. When the kidneys are damaged or fail to function properly, waste products can build up in the body, leading to many symptoms and complications, including high blood pressure, anemia, bone disease, and nerve damage.

Adopting a renal-friendly diet is one of the most critical steps toward managing kidney disease or other renal issues. A renal diet is an eating plan to help support kidney health and prevent further kidney damage. This diet typically involves reducing the intake of certain nutrients, such as sodium, phosphorus, and protein, while increasing the intake of other nutrients, such as fiber and healthy fats.

However, for many, the idea of a "renal diet" may seem overwhelming, restrictive, and tasteless. If you are struggling with renal issues, you are not alone. The good news is that plenty of delicious and nutritious foods can support your kidney health and help you feel your best. And that is where this Renal Diet Cookbook comes in.

In the following chapters, you will find easy-to-follow recipes for kidney health. Whether you are looking for hearty main dishes, satisfying snacks, or sweet treats, we have got you covered. By following the recipes in this book, you will learn how to make flavorful meals that meet your dietary needs without sacrificing taste.

Not only will this renal diet cookbook help you eat more healthily, but it will also help you feel more confident in the kitchen. We want to show you that a renal diet can be delicious and enjoyable and that you do not have to give up your favorite foods to maintain your kidney health.

The recipes in this cookbook have been carefully selected and tested to ensure they meet the nutritional needs of people with renal issues. They are based on the principles of a renal diet, which emphasizes the importance of limiting sodium, phosphorus, and protein intake while increasing the intake of fiber and healthy fats.

Some of the key ingredients that you will find in many of the recipes in this book include fresh fruits and vegetables, whole grains, lean proteins, and low-fat dairy products. These ingredients are kidney-friendly and packed with nutrients supporting overall health and well-being.

In addition to the recipes, this book also includes information on the principles of a renal diet, meal planning tips, preparation tips, and guidance on making healthy food choices for kidney health. Whether you are new to the renal diet or have been following it for years, this book is a valuable resource for anyone looking to improve their kidney health through healthy and delicious food choices.

By incorporating the recipes in this book into your meal plan, you can manage your renal issues and support your overall health and well-being. A renal diet can effectively manage kidney disease, reduce the risk of complications, and improve quality of life.

So, let us get started on this culinary journey toward a healthier and happier life. In Chapter 1, we will begin with some basic information on renal diets and how to make healthy food choices for kidney health.

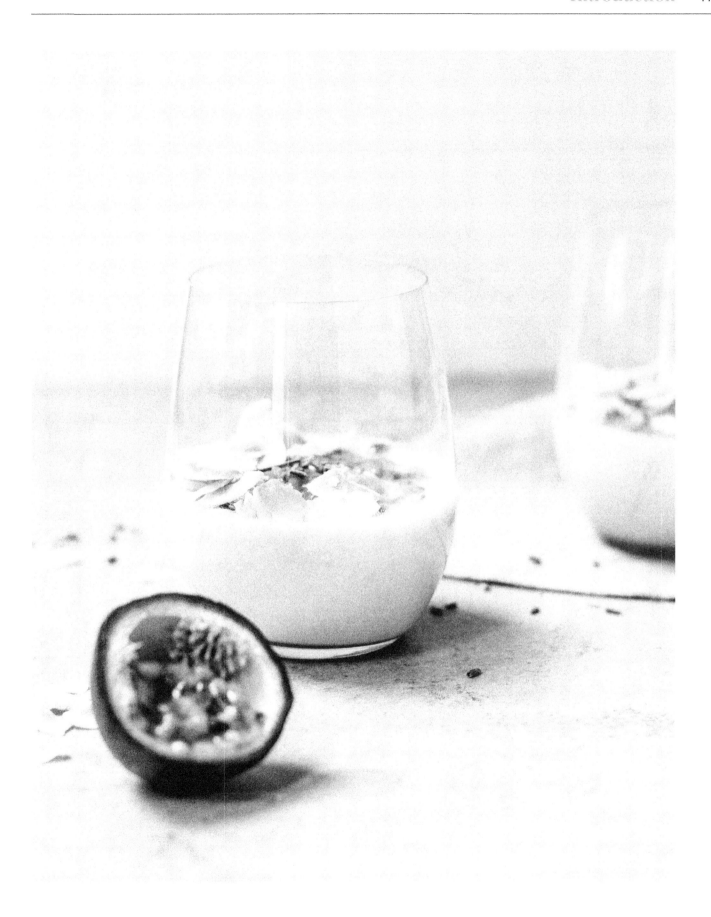

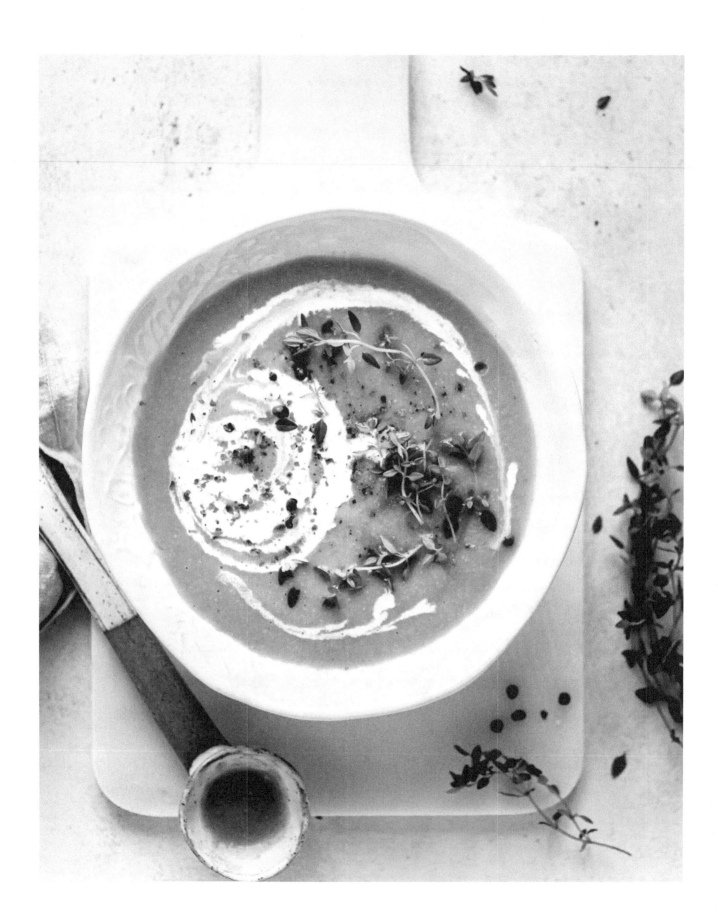

Chapter 1 WHAT IS RENAL DISEASE?

The kidneys are essential for filtering waste and excess fluids from the blood, regulating electrolyte levels, and producing hormones that control red blood cell production and blood pressure. However, when the kidneys become damaged or diseased, they may not function properly, leading to a build up of fluids and waste in the body.

The kidneys are like a delicate ecosystem; when one part breaks down, it can have a ripple effect on the whole system. Understanding renal disease is the first step towards managing its symptoms and adopting healthy dietary and lifestyle habits to preserve kidney function.

In this chapter, we will explore the basics of renal disease, focusing on chronic kidney disease (CKD), its stages, causes, symptoms, and other forms of renal disease.

INTRODUCTION TO RENAL DISEASE

ANY DISEASE THAT AFFECTS THE KIDNEYS' STRUCTURE OR FUNCTION, IMPAIRING THEIR CAPACITY TO EFFECTIVELY FILTER WASTE AND EXTRA FLUID FROM THE BLOOD IS REFERRED TO AS A RENAL DISEASE.

Renal disease is often known as kidney disease. The kidneys are vital organs that perform essential tasks to sustain overall health. The kidneys' main job is to maintain the proper balance of electrolytes like salt and potassium and filter out waste materials and extra fluid from the blood.

Renal disease may be a challenge, but it does not define us. We are more than our diagnosis. People of various ages and races can develop renal disease, ranging from mild to severe. Chronic kidney disease (CKD), which affects millions of individuals globally, is the most prevalent renal illness. CKD, a long-term, progressive disorder, can result in irreparable kidney damage if left untreated. Acute kidney damage, another type of renal disease, is a sudden occurrence that various causes, including injuries, drugs, and infections, can set on.

Renal disease can have a range of causes, including high blood pressure, diabetes, infections, autoimmune disorders, and genetic conditions. Risk factors for renal disease may include age, ethnicity, family history, obesity, and smoking.

The symptoms of renal disease may differ depending on the underlying cause and intensity of the condition. There may be no noticeable symptoms in the preliminary stages of kidney disease, and kidney function may only be slightly reduced. As the disease progresses, however, symptoms such as fatigue, nausea, swelling, changes in urination, and other complications may occur.

Early diagnosis and treatment of renal disease are crucial to managing the condition and preventing further kidney damage. Treatment may involve medications, lifestyle changes, and, in severe cases, dialysis or kidney transplantation.

CHRONIC KIDNEY DISEASE (CKD)

CKD stands for chronic kidney disease. It is a long-term condition in which the kidneys gradually lose their ability to function correctly over time. CKD is a common and severe condition affecting millions worldwide and is a leading cause of morbidity and mortality. The illness is characterized by a gradual and steady decline in kidney function over months or years, which causes the body to swell with waste materials and fluids.

The early stages of CKD may have no noticeable symptoms, and the condition may be diagnosed through routine blood and urine tests. As the disease progresses, symptoms such as fatigue, nausea, vomiting, and changes in urination may occur. Complications of CKD can include high blood pressure, bone disease, anemia, and cardiovascular disease.

CKD is typically diagnosed based on a combination of blood and urine tests, which can measure kidney function, estimate the level of kidney damage, and detect any underlying conditions or complications. Treatment for CKD may involve medications to manage blood pressure and other complications, lifestyle changes such as diet and exercise, and, in severe cases, dialysis or kidney transplantation.

CAUSES AND SYMPTOMS OF CKD

Chronic kidney disease (CKD) can have a variety of causes, including high blood pressure, diabetes, polycystic kidney disease, glomerulonephritis, and other inherited or acquired conditions. In some cases, the reasons may be unknown. Understanding the underlying cause of CKD is essential in developing an effective treatment plan and preventing further kidney damage.

CAUSES OF CKD

Diabetes is the leading cause of kidney disease in the United States. High blood pressure is the second leading cause. Other causes of CKD may include:

- Glomerulonephritis (GN) is a condition that damages the kidneys' filtering units.

- Polycystic kidney disease is a genetic disorder that causes cysts to form in the kidneys.
- Other inherited or acquired conditions that can damage the kidneys over time.

Risk factors for developing CKD include age, family history of kidney disease, obesity, smoking, and a history of kidney stones. Certain medications and toxins, including nonsteroidal anti-inflammatory drugs and heavy metals, can also harm the kidneys and lead to CKD.

SYMPTOMS OF CKD

There may be no noticeable symptoms in the early stages of kidney disease. As the CKD progresses, symptoms may include fatigue, weakness, vomiting, nausea, loss of appetite, changes in urination, swelling in the hands and feet, and difficulty concentrating. In severe cases, CKD can cause anemia, bone disease, high blood pressure, and cardiovascular disease. It is important to note that other conditions can cause many non-specific symptoms. Therefore, it is essential to undergo routine blood and urine tests to screen for CKD, especially if you have risk factors for the disease or are experiencing any of the symptoms mentioned above.

In the next section of this chapter, we will discuss how CKD is diagnosed and the tests used to monitor kidney function.

DIAGNOSING AND MONITORING CKD

Early detection and monitoring of CKD are crucial to slowing the progression of the disease and preventing complications. Routine blood and urine tests are used to screen for CKD, especially in individuals with risk factors, such as diabetes, high blood pressure, or a family history of kidney disease.

DIAGNOSING CKD

A diagnosis of CKD is made based on kidney damage or decreased renal function that lasts for three or more months. Kidney damage may be indicated by blood or protein in the urine. In contrast, reduced kidney function may be characterized by a decrease in the glomerular filtration rate (GFR), a measure of how efficiently the kidneys filter waste products from the blood.

To diagnose CKD, your healthcare provider may perform the following tests:

▶ IMAGING TESTS:

Imaging tests such as ultrasound or CT scan may be used to evaluate the kidneys and surrounding structures.

▶ BLOOD TESTS:
A blood test called serum creatinine is used to estimate the GFR. Other blood tests may be used to assess overall kidney function and monitor for complications of CKD, such as anemia or high potassium levels.

▶ URINE TESTS:
A urine test called a urinalysis looks for protein or blood in the urine.

MONITORING CKD

Once a diagnosis of CKD has been made, ongoing monitoring is necessary to assess kidney function and monitor for complications. The frequency of monitoring may vary depending on the severity of the disease, but it typically involves regular blood and urine tests.

In addition to urine and blood tests, other measures may be taken to monitor the progression of CKD and prevent complications. For example, blood pressure control is essential in individuals with CKD, as high blood pressure can further damage the kidneys. Medications may be prescribed to lower the risk of cardiovascular disease and control blood pressure.

In some cases, individuals with CKD may need to modify their diet to help manage the disease. An expert dietitian can help develop a personalized meal plan. It will consider the individual's nutritional needs and helps manage CKD.

STAGES OF CKD

Understanding the stages of CKD is crucial in managing the condition and making informed decisions about treatment options, including adopting a renal diet and lifestyle.

CKD is a progressive disease classified into five stages depending on the level of renal function. The stages are determined based on the glomerular filtration rate (GFR), which measures how well the kidneys perform. The lower the GFR, the more severe the renal disease.

▶ STAGE 1: KIDNEY DAMAGE WITH NORMAL OR HIGH GFR
In stage 1 of CKD, there is evidence of kidney damage, but the GFR is high or normal (GFR ≥ 90 mL/min). This phase is often called "kidney damage with normal or mildly reduced GFR" and may not cause symptoms.

► STAGE 2: KIDNEY DAMAGE WITH MILDLY REDUCED GFR

In stage 2 of CKD, there is evidence of renal damage and a mildly reduced GFR (GFR = 60 to 89 mL/min). This is often called "kidney damage with mildly reduced GFR" and may not cause symptoms.

► STAGE 3: MODERATE DECREASE IN GFR

Stage 3 of renal disease is divided into two sub-stages: stage 3a & step 3b. In the first one (3a), the GFR is moderately decreased (GFR = 45 to 59 mL/min), while in the second stage (3b), the GFR is severely reduced (GFR between 30 & 44 mL/min). Individuals with stage 3 CKD may experience symptoms such as fatigue, fluid retention, and changes in urine output.

► STAGE 4: SEVERE DECREASE IN GFR

In stage 4 of CKD, there is a severe decrease in glomerular filtration rate (GFR = 15 to 29 mL/min). Individuals with stage 4 CKD may experience fatigue, fluid retention, anemia, and bone disease.

► STAGE 5: KIDNEY FAILURE

Stage 5 of CKD, also known as end-stage renal disease, occurs when the glomerular filtration rate is less (GFR < 15 mL/min). At this phase, the kidneys are no longer able to function correctly. Such individuals require dialysis or a kidney transplant to stay alive.

It is vital to note that CKD is a progressive disease that can worsen over time if not appropriately managed. However, early detection and management can slow the progression of this issue and improve your overall health.

OTHER FORMS OF RENAL DISEASE

CKD is the most common form of renal disease, but other kidney disorders can affect kidney function and health. These may include kidney infections, kidney stones, and genetic disorders like polycystic kidney disease. Proper diagnosis and treatment of these conditions are essential to managing kidney health and preventing further damage.

► GLOMERULONEPHRITIS

This is a group of diseases that cause inflammation of the glomeruli. Glomeruli are tiny filters in the kidneys that remove waste and excess fluids from the blood. This inflammation can damage the kidneys and lead to CKD.

► NEPHROTIC SYNDROME

This group of symptoms occurs when the kidneys leak large amounts of protein into the urine, leading to swelling and fluid retention. Various underlying conditions, including glomerulonephritis and diabetes, can cause nephrotic syndrome.

► ACUTE KIDNEY INJURY

AKI is a sudden and temporary loss of renal function due to injury, infection, medication use, or other causes. AKI is typically reversible, but it can lead to chronic renal disease if not managed properly.

► URINARY TRACT INFECTIONS

UTIs are infections that occur in the urinary system, including the kidneys, bladder, and urethra. If left untreated, UTIs can cause inflammation and kidney damage, leading to CKD.

► POLYCYSTIC KIDNEY DISEASE

PKD is a genetic disorder that causes fluid-filled cysts to form in the kidneys, eventually leading to kidney failure. PKD can also cause cysts in other organs, such as the liver.

It is important to note that the treatment for these other forms of renal disease may differ from the treatment for CKD. Individuals with these conditions should work closely with their healthcare team to manage their condition effectively.

CHAPTER SUMMARY

Renal disease is a severe condition that affects the functioning of the kidneys, which are vital organs responsible for filtering waste products from the blood. Several types of renal disease can have various symptoms and complications that can impact a person's overall health and well-being.

Individuals with CKD or other kidney issues must understand the importance of managing their condition through lifestyle modifications such as diet, exercise, and medication. Making healthy choices and following a renal-friendly diet can help support kidney health and prevent further damage.

People who are already healthy don't always benefit much from this diet. But if you have hypertension or suspect salt sensitivity, DASH may be an excellent solution.

IN THE NEXT CHAPTER, WE WILL DISCUSS THE ROLE OF DIET IN MANAGING CKD AND THE SPECIFIC DIETARY GUIDELINES THAT INDIVIDUALS WITH CKD SHOULD FOLLOW.

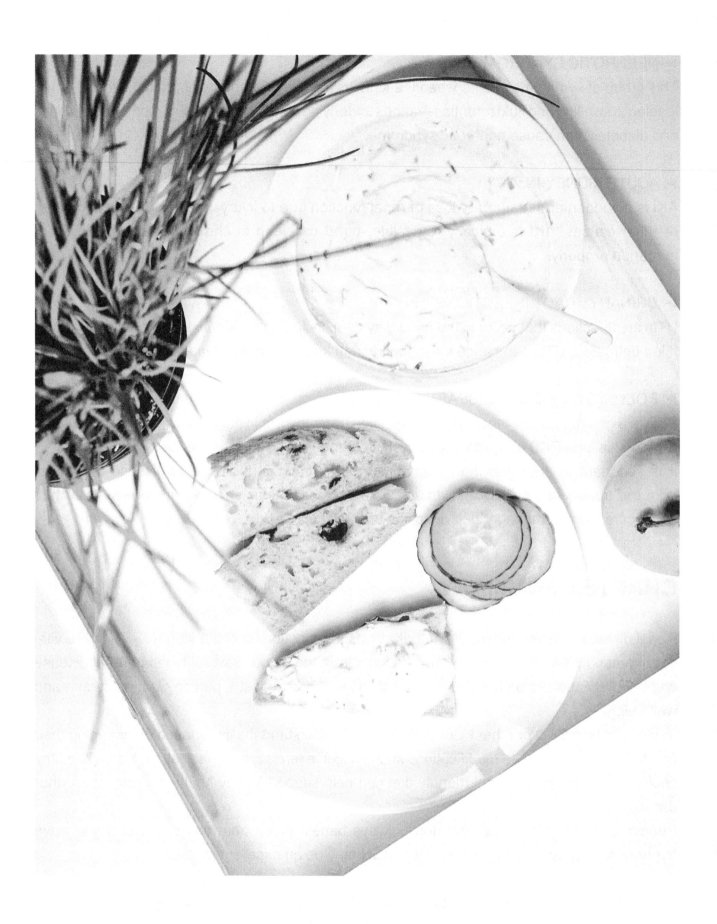

Chapter 2

RENAL DIET

The major benefits of the Renal diet

Understanding macronutrients in the Renal diet

Meal planning and preparation tips or a Renal diet

LIVING WITH RENAL DISEASE IS A JOURNEY, NOT A DESTINATION. IT REQUIRES PATIENCE, PERSEVERANCE, AND A LOT OF SELF-CARE..

Managing chronic kidney disease (CKD) requires a multifaceted approach that includes medication, exercise, and diet modification. This chapter will focus on the renal diet and its role in managing kidney diseases. The renal diet is a specific eating plan designed to help preserve renal function and slow the progression of CKD. It involves limiting certain nutrients that can stress the kidneys while ensuring that individuals with CKD still get the necessary nutrients to maintain overall health.

In this chapter, we will discuss the renal diet and its significant benefits and offer tips and warnings to help individuals with CKD navigate this critical aspect of their treatment plan.

THE MAJOR BENEFITS OF THE RENAL DIET

The renal diet is an eating plan that can benefit individuals with kidney diseases. The following are some of the significant benefits of the renal diet:

▶ REDUCES STRESS ON THE KIDNEYS
The renal diet aims to reduce the number of waste products and fluids the kidneys have to filter. By limiting certain nutrients, such as sodium, potassium, and phosphorus, the diet can help reduce the workload on the kidneys and slow the progression of kidney disease.

▶ OPTIMIZE BLOOD PRESSURE
High blood pressure is a common issue of CKD. The renal diet focuses on reducing sodium intake. This step can assist lower blood pressure and minimize the risk of heart disease.

▶ CONTROLS BLOOD SUGAR LEVELS
The renal diet also emphasizes the importance of controlling blood sugar levels, particularly for individuals with diabetes, who are at a higher risk of developing kidney diseases. The diet encourages limiting foods high in simple sugars and refined carbohydrates, which can cause spikes in blood sugar levels.

▶ MAINTAINS PROPER NUTRITION
While the renal diet restricts certain nutrients, it also emphasizes the importance of adequate

protein, vitamins, and minerals. This ensures that individuals with CKD still get the necessary nutrients to maintain overall health.

▶ IMPROVES OVERALL HEALTH OUTCOMES

By reducing stress on the kidneys and managing other health conditions, such as diabetes, and high blood pressure, the renal diet can improve overall health outcomes for individuals with CKD. Studies have shown that following the renal diet can improve quality of life, improve physical functioning, and reduce mortality risk.

UNDERSTANDING MACRONUTRIENTS IN THE RENAL DIET

Macronutrients, which include carbohydrates, proteins, and fats, are essential components of any diet, including the renal diet. However, in the renal diet, it is vital to focus on the quantity and quality of these macronutrients, as the kidneys may not be able to handle excessive amounts of certain nutrients. Here is a breakdown of each macronutrient and its role in the renal diet:

▶ CARBOHYDRATES

These are the body's primary energy source, but some carbohydrates can harm individuals with CKD. Simple carbohydrates, such as sugar and refined grains, should be limited. The reason is that:

- They can cause spikes in blood sugar levels. They can also increase the risk of complications such as diabetes.

Complex carbohydrates, such as whole grains, fruits, and vegetables, are a better choice as they are digested more slowly and provide a steady energy source.

▶ PROTEINS

Protein is essential for building and repairing tissues, but excess protein can stress the kidneys. Therefore, individuals with kidney disease need to limit their protein intake. The recommended daily protein intake for individuals with CKD varies depending on the stage of the disease, but it generally ranges from 0.6 to 0.8 grams per kilogram of body weight. Lean meats, poultry, fish, eggs, and dairy products are high-quality protein sources. These are preferred over lower-quality sources, such as processed meats and plant-based protein substitutes.

▶ FATS

Fats provide energy, help absorb specific vitamins, and contribute to the flavor and texture of foods. However, it is essential to limit the intake of certain types of fat, such as saturated and trans fats. They can increase the risk of heart disease. Healthy fats, such as monounsaturated and polyunsaturated fats, are a better choice and can be found in nuts, seeds, fatty fish, and avocados. The renal diet emphasizes the importance of paying attention to the quantity and quality of macronutrients. Limiting simple carbohydrates, moderating protein intake, and choosing healthy fats can help individuals with CKD maintain proper nutrition while reducing kidney stress. Consulting with a registered dietitian specializing in renal food can also help develop a personalized renal diet plan.

MEAL PLANNING AND PREPARATION TIPS FOR A RENAL DIET

Planning and preparing meals for a renal diet can be challenging, but it can become a manageable task with some simple tips and strategies. Here are some critical tips for meal planning and preparation for a renal diet:

▶ PLAN YOUR MEALS

Planning meals ahead of time can save time and reduce stress. Make a weekly meal plan and grocery list to help you stay on track.

▶ LIMIT SODIUM INTAKE

Sodium is a mineral that can harm the kidneys when consumed in excess. Be mindful of high-sodium foods and opt for low-sodium alternatives when possible.

▶ MONITOR PORTION SIZES

Overeating any food can be harmful to the kidneys. Monitoring portion sizes can help ensure the right amount of nutrients are consumed without overloading the kidneys.

▶ CHOOSE LEAN PROTEIN SOURCES

Protein is an essential nutrient, but too much protein can stress the kidneys. Choose lean protein sources like chicken, fish, and lean cuts of beef, and avoid processed meats.

▶ EXPERIMENT WITH NEW RECIPES

A renal diet can become repetitive if the same meals are consumed repeatedly. Try new recipes and experiment with different flavors to keep meals interesting.

▶ INCORPORATE LOW-POTASSIUM FRUITS & VEGETABLES

Fruits and vegetables are vital components of a healthy diet but can also be high in potassium. Incorporate low-potassium options like berries, grapes, and green beans into meals to minimize the risk of potassium build up in the blood.

▶ USE HERBS AND SPICES INSTEAD OF SALT

Salt is a common seasoning that can harm the kidneys when consumed excessively. Instead, try using herbs and spices to add flavor to meals.

▶ PREP MEALS IN ADVANCE

Prepping meals in advance can save time and make meal times less stressful. Consider batch cooking and storing meals in the freezer for easy reheating later.

CHAPTER SUMMARY

The renal diet is essential to managing kidney disease and other kidney-related issues. It focuses on reducing the intake of certain nutrients that can strain the kidneys while ensuring that the body receives adequate nutrition.

Individuals can manage their condition effectively and prevent further complications by following a renal diet. However, it is important to note that everyone's nutritional needs may vary based on their health status and stage of kidney disease.

MEAL PLANNING AND PREPARATION FOR A RENAL DIET CAN TAKE SOME TIME AND EFFORT, BUT IT CAN BECOME A MANAGEABLE TASK WITH THE RIGHT STRATEGIES IN PLACE.

THE NEXT CHAPTER WILL DELVE INTO THE SPECIFIC NUTRIENTS ESSENTIAL FOR REGULATING KIDNEY FUNCTION, SUCH AS POTASSIUM, PHOSPHORUS, AND SODIUM. READ ON!

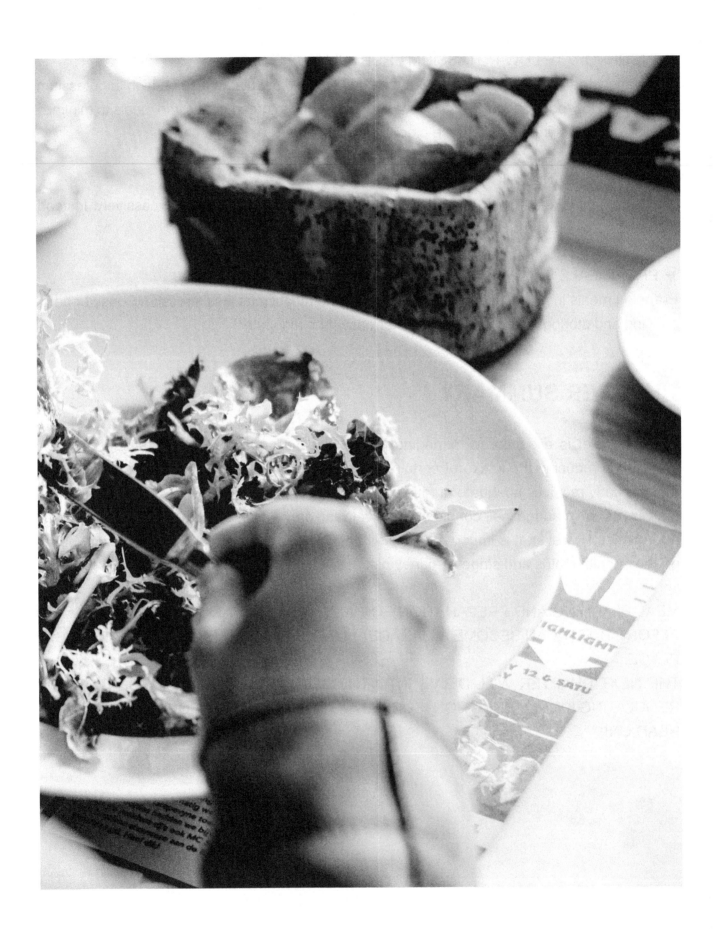

WHAT NUTRIENTS DO I NEED TO REGULATE?

Chapter 3

Sodium: The Silent Killer

Potassium: To Limit or Not to Limit?

The Importance of Protein in the Renal Diet

Fats: The Good & The Bad

Fruits and Vegetables: Friend or Foe?

The Role of Beverages and Juice in the Renal Diet

Foods to Avoid on a Renal Diet

Your diet is crucial to managing your condition if you have renal disease. A healthy renal diet requires regulating certain nutrients, such as sodium, potassium, and fats, to prevent further kidney damage and promote overall health. By understanding the role of these nutrients in your diet, you can take control of your health and manage your renal disease effectively.

THIS CHAPTER WILL DISCUSS THE NUTRIENTS THAT NEED TO BE REGULATED IN A RENAL DIET, WHY THEY ARE ESSENTIAL, AND HOW TO MONITOR AND CONTROL THEM.

SODIUM: THE SILENT KILLER

Sodium is an essential mineral found in salt that our body requires for various functions such as regulating blood pressure, transmitting nerve impulses, and balancing fluids. However, sodium intake needs to be strictly monitored and controlled for people with renal disease. High sodium intake can cause fluid build up, leading to increased blood pressure, swelling, and potential kidney damage.

The recommended daily sodium intake for a healthy individual is 2,300 milligrams (mg), but the limit is much lower for people with renal disease, usually around 1,500-2,000 mg per day. Sodium is present in almost all processed and packaged foods, including canned soups, frozen dinners, and even breakfast cereals. Therefore, reading food labels carefully and choosing low-sodium alternatives whenever possible is essential.

▶ TIPS FOR REDUCING SODIUM INTAKE

1. Some tips for reducing sodium intake in a renal diet include:
2. Limiting the use of salt and salt-based seasonings in cooking.
3. Using spices and herbs to add flavor to food instead of salt.
4. Choosing fresh or frozen fruits and vegetables instead of canned ones.
5. Avoiding processed and packaged foods as much as possible.
6. Rinsing canned foods like beans and vegetables before consuming to reduce the sodium content.

Monitoring and controlling sodium intake is an essential aspect of a renal diet. Reducing sodium intake can help manage your blood pressure and reduce fluid build up, protecting your kidneys from further damage.

POTASSIUM: TO LIMIT OR NOT TO LIMIT?

Potassium is a mineral found in many foods that we eat. It is essential for regulating the heartbeat, maintaining normal blood pressure, and keeping our muscles and nerves functioning correctly. However, excess potassium in the blood can be dangerous and even life-threatening for people with kidney disease. Therefore, monitoring and regulating potassium intake for individuals with kidney disease is essential.

▶ POTASSIUM AND KIDNEY DISEASE

The kidneys filter potassium from the blood and remove it through urine. When the kidneys are not functioning correctly, potassium can build up in the bloodstream, leading to hyperkalemia. Symptoms of hyperkalemia may include weakness, nausea, and an irregular heartbeat, which can be life-threatening.

▶ POTASSIUM REQUIREMENTS

The amount of potassium an individual with kidney disease can consume will depend on the stage of their condition. In the early phases of kidney disease, individuals may not need to limit their potassium intake. However, potassium intake should be defined as kidney function declines to prevent hyperkalemia. The recommended potassium intake for individuals with kidney disease can range from 2,000 to 3,000 milligrams per day.

▶ POTASSIUM-RICH FOODS

Foods high in potassium (K) include potatoes, bananas, tomatoes, avocados, spinach, and oranges. These foods should be eaten in moderation or avoided entirely by individuals with kidney disease. Discussing a personalized meal plan with a dietitian is essential.

▶ POTASSIUM BINDERS

In some cases, individuals with kidney disease may need to take potassium binders, medications that bind to potassium in the digestive tract and prevent its absorption. These medications can help lower potassium levels in the blood and avoid hyperkalemia. However, potassium binders can also have side effects, such as constipation, and should only be taken under the guidance of a healthcare provider.

Monitoring and regulating potassium intake is essential for individuals with kidney disease to prevent hyperkalemia and other complications. Individuals can meet their nutritional needs by working with an expert and following a personalized meal plan while maintaining safe potassium levels.

THE IMPORTANCE OF PROTEIN IN THE RENAL DIET

Protein is essential for maintaining good health in individuals with renal disease. It is vital to consume enough protein to maintain muscle mass, prevent muscle wasting, and promote overall well-being. However, individuals with the renal disease must be cautious about their protein intake and understand the importance of including high-quality protein sources in their renal diet.

▶ THE ROLE OF PROTEIN IN THE BODY

Protein is an essential macronutrient that is vital in building and repairing tissues. It is also helpful for producing enzymes and hormones and maintaining fluid balance in the body. It is also a significant source of energy for the body.

▶ THE IMPORTANCE OF PROTEIN IN THE RENAL DIET

Individuals with renal disease often experience a decline in kidney function, which can result in the accumulation of waste in the body. This can lead to a condition called uremia, which can cause various health problems, including muscle wasting. Adequate protein intake is critical in preventing muscle loss and maintaining overall health in individuals with renal disease.

▶ THE RECOMMENDED DAILY PROTEIN INTAKE

The recommended daily protein intake for individuals with renal disease varies based on the stage of the disease and other factors such as age, gender, and physical activity level. A registered dietitian can help determine an individual's specific protein needs based on their unique circumstances.

▶ HIGH-QUALITY PROTEIN SOURCES

Individuals with the renal disease must include high-quality protein sources, such as lean meats, poultry, fish, and eggs. Plant-based protein sources such as beans, lentils, and tofu are also good options. However, individuals with renal disease should limit their intake of high-potassium plant-based protein sources such as soy products and legumes.

► PROTEIN SUPPLEMENTS AND RENAL DISEASE

Protein supplements such as whey and casein are popular among athletes and bodybuilders. However, individuals with renal disease should be cautious when using these supplements, as they can place additional stress on the kidneys. It is always best to consult a healthcare provider before using dietary supplements.

Protein is an essential nutrient that is critical in maintaining overall health. However, individuals with renal disease must be cautious about their protein intake and ensure they consume high-quality protein sources in their renal diet. A registered dietitian can help determine an individual's specific protein needs and develop a customized renal diet plan that meets their unique nutritional requirements.

FATS: THE GOOD & THE BAD

Fats are essential nutrients that play a vital role in the body, but not all fats are created equal. Understanding the difference between good and bad fats is necessary for individuals with renal disease to maintain optimal health. Including good sources of fat in the renal diet and limiting the intake of bad fats is also an essential aspect of a healthy renal diet.

► THE ROLE OF FATS IN THE BODY

Fats are an essential macronutrient that plays a vital role in the body's energy production, insulation, and cushioning of organs. Fats also help in the absorption of fat-soluble vitamins.

► TYPES OF FATS

There are three types of fats. These include saturated, unsaturated, and trans fats.

1. **Saturated**
   - These are solid at room temperature. They are found in animal products such as meat, butter, cheese, and cream.
   - Saturated fats are considered bad fats because they can increase the risk of heart disease and raise cholesterol levels in the blood.

2. Unsaturated

- These are liquid at room temperature. They are found in plant-based oils such as olive, canola, and nuts.
- Unsaturated fats are considered good because they can reduce the risk of heart and lower cholesterol levels in the blood.

3. Trans

- These are formed when unsaturated fats are hydrogenated to make them solid at room temperature.
- These are usually found in processed foods such as baked goods, margarine, and fast food.
- They are considered the worst type of fats as they raise harmful cholesterol levels in the blood and increase the risk of heart disease.

▶ THE IMPORTANCE OF FATS IN THE RENAL DIET

Fats are an essential nutrient that should be included in the renal diet, but choosing suitable fats is crucial. Individuals with renal disease should limit their intake of trans and saturated fats and choose unsaturated fats instead.

GOOD SOURCES OF FATS IN THE RENAL DIET:
Good sources of fats in the renal diet include fatty fish such as nuts and seeds, salmon and tuna, avocado, and plant-based oils such as olive and canola.

HOW TO LIMIT BAD FATS IN THE RENAL DIET
Understanding the importance of good fats and limiting the intake of bad fats is crucial for individuals with renal disease to maintain optimal health. Incorporating a healthy balance of fats in the renal diet can improve health outcomes and quality of life.
Individuals with renal disease should avoid processed foods, fried foods, and fatty meats to limit the intake of bad fats. It is also important to read food labels and look for products low in trans and saturated fats.

FRUITS AND VEGETABLES: FRIEND OR FOE?

Fruits and vegetables are crucial parts of a healthy diet. Still, for individuals with renal disease, it is essential to understand which fruits and vegetables are safe to consume in moderation.

▶ THE BENEFITS OF FRUITS & VEGETABLES

Fruits and vegetables are packed with essential vitamins, minerals, and antioxidants. These can help reduce inflammation, lower blood pressure, and prevent chronic diseases like cancer and heart disease.

THE ROLE OF FRUITS AND VEGETABLES IN THE RENAL DIET

The renal diet should include fruits and vegetables to provide essential nutrients and fiber. However, some fruits and vegetables may be high in potassium and phosphorus, harming individuals with renal disease.

- High-potassium fruits & vegetables

High-potassium fruits and vegetables that should be limited in the renal diet include bananas, oranges, kiwis, melons, tomatoes, avocados, and leafy greens such as spinach and kale.

- Low-potassium fruits & vegetables

Low-potassium fruits and vegetables that are safe to consume in moderation include apples, berries, grapes, peaches, pears, green beans, carrots, and cauliflower.

- High-phosphorus fruits & vegetables

High-phosphorus fruits and vegetables that should be limited in the renal diet include dried fruits, such as raisins and dates, nuts, and seeds.

- Low-phosphorus fruits & vegetables

Low-phosphorus fruits and vegetables that are safe to consume in moderation include strawberries, blueberries, raspberries, cherries, cabbage, and cucumbers.

▶ THE IMPORTANCE OF PORTION CONTROL

While fruits and vegetables are essential to a healthy diet, individuals with renal disease should consume them in moderation to avoid consuming too much potassium and phosphorus.

Fruits and vegetables are an essential part of a healthy diet. Still, for individuals with renal disease, it is necessary to be mindful of which fruits and vegetables are safe to consume in moderation.

HIGH-POTASSIUM AND HIGH-PHOSPHORUS FRUITS AND VEGETABLES SHOULD BE LIMITED, WHILE LOW-POTASSIUM AND LOW-PHOSPHORUS FRUITS AND VEGETABLES CAN BE INCLUDED IN THE RENAL DIET IN MODERATION..

Practicing portion control is also essential to avoid consuming too much potassium and phosphorus. Incorporating a variety of fruits and vegetables into the renal diet can provide essential nutrients and fiber while promoting optimal health outcomes.

THE ROLE OF BEVERAGES AND JUICE IN THE RENAL DIET

Beverages and juices can play an essential role in the renal diet, but choosing beverages wisely and consuming them in moderation is vital. Water is the best choice for hydration, while sugary and alcoholic drinks should be avoided. Freshly squeezed juices can provide essential nutrients but should be consumed cautiously due to their potassium and sugar content. Smoothies can be a healthy way to consume fruits and vegetables, but they should be made with low-potassium ingredients and consumed in moderation. However, it is essential to be mindful of the types and amounts of beverages and juices consumed, as some may be high in sodium, potassium, or phosphorus.

▶ BEVERAGES TO AVOID OR LIMIT

- Sugary beverages, such as soda, sports drinks, and energy drinks, can be high in calories and added sugars, contributing to high blood sugar levels and weight gain.
- Caffeinated beverages like coffee and tea can dehydrate and increase blood pressure if consumed excessively.
- Alcoholic beverages can harm the kidneys and should be avoided or limited.

▶ BEVERAGES TO CONSUME IN MODERATION

- Low-sodium broths and soups can provide hydration and essential nutrients, such as protein and minerals, but should be consumed in moderation due to their sodium content.
- Herbal teas and decaf coffee can be hydrating and provide antioxidants but should be consumed in moderation.
- Freshly squeezed juices can provide essential vitamins and minerals but should be consumed in moderation due to their potassium and sugar content.

► THE IMPORTANCE OF HYDRATION

- Individuals with kidney disease may have difficulty filtering and excreting excess fluid, leading to edema or fluid build up in the body.
- Adequate hydration can help prevent dehydration, improve kidney function, and flush out excess waste and fluid.
- Water is the best choice for hydration, as it contains no added sugars, sodium, or calories.

► THE ROLE OF JUICE IN THE RENAL DIET

- Freshly squeezed juices can be a healthy addition to the renal diet but should be consumed cautiously.
- Certain juices, such as orange and tomato juice, can be high in potassium and should be limited or avoided.
- Low-potassium juices, such as apple and cranberry juice, can be consumed in moderation.

► THE ROLE OF SMOOTHIES IN THE RENAL DIET

- Smoothies can be a healthy and convenient way to consume fruits and vegetables, but they should be made with low-potassium ingredients and in moderation.
- Adding protein sources, such as Greek yogurt or whey protein powder, can help promote satiety and provide essential nutrients.

FOODS TO AVOID ON A RENAL DIET

A renal diet is designed to help manage kidney disease and prevent further kidney damage. Individuals with kidney disease must avoid certain foods that can harm the kidneys or contribute to other health problems. Below are some common foods to avoid on a renal diet:

► HIGH-SODIUM FOODS

- Sodium can contribute to high blood pressure, further damaging the kidneys.
- Processed and packaged food should be avoided or consumed in moderation (such as frozen dinners, canned soups, and snacks).
- Table salt and seasonings containing salt, such as garlic and onion, should be avoided or limited.

- Fast and restaurant meals are often high in sodium and should be avoided or limited.

▶ HIGH-POTASSIUM FOODS

- Our kidneys play a vital role in regulating potassium levels in the body, and individuals with kidney disease may have difficulty excreting excess potassium.
- High-potassium foods should be limited or avoided (such as bananas, oranges, tomatoes, potatoes, and avocados).
- Salt substitutes that contain potassium should also be avoided.

▶ HIGH-PHOSPHORUS FOODS

- The kidneys play an essential role in regulating phosphorus levels in the body, and individuals with kidney disease may have difficulty excreting excess phosphorus.
- High-phosphorus foods should be limited or avoided (such as dairy products, nuts, seeds, and certain types of fish).
- Processed and packaged foods, such as soda, baked goods, and processed meats, may also be high in phosphorus and should be avoided or limited.

▶ HIGH-PROTEIN FOODS

- Protein is an essential nutrient for the body but consuming too much protein can harm the kidneys.
- High-protein foods should be consumed in moderation (such as red meat, poultry, fish, and eggs).
- Plant-based protein sources, such as legumes, tofu, and tempeh, can be a healthy alternative to animal-based protein sources.

▶ FOODS WITH ADDED SUGARS

- Consuming too much sugar can contribute to high blood sugar levels and weight gain, which can further damage the kidneys
- Foods with added sugars should be limited or avoided (such as candy, soda, and baked goods)
- Natural sweeteners, such as honey and maple syrup, can be used in moderation

Individuals with the renal disease must work with an expert to develop a personalized renal diet plan considering their nutrient needs and health goals. In addition to avoiding certain foods, it is also essential to consume a variety of nutrient-rich foods, such as vegetables, fruits, whole grains, and lean protein sources, to support overall health and kidney function.

CHAPTER SUMMARY

For individuals with renal or kidney disease, it is vital to regulate certain nutrients in their diet to manage their condition and prevent further kidney damage. The nutrients that need to be controlled on a renal diet include:

- Fluids: Fluid intake should be monitored and limited to prevent fluid build up in the body, which can strain the kidneys.
- Protein: Individuals with kidney disease may need to limit their protein intake to reduce the workload on their kidneys.
- Vitamin D & calcium: These nutrients may need to be supplemented to maintain healthy bones and prevent bone disease.
- Sodium: Sodium intake should be limited to control blood pressure and reduce the risk of fluid build up in the body.
- Phosphorus: Phosphorus intake should be limited to prevent bone disease and mineral imbalances in the body.
- Potassium: Individuals with kidney disease may need to limit their potassium intake to prevent dangerous potassium levels in the blood.

Working with a healthcare professional to create a personalized renal diet plan that meets individual needs and restrictions is essential. A well-balanced and regulated renal diet can help manage kidney disease and improve overall health.

NOW THAT WE HAVE DISCUSSED THE IMPORTANCE OF A BALANCED DIET AND REGULATING CERTAIN NUTRIENTS FOR OPTIMAL HEALTH, WE WILL EXPLORE THE BENEFITS OF EXERCISE AND PHYSICAL ACTIVITY FOR OVERALL WELL-BEING IN THE NEXT CHAPTER.

* * * * * * * * * * *

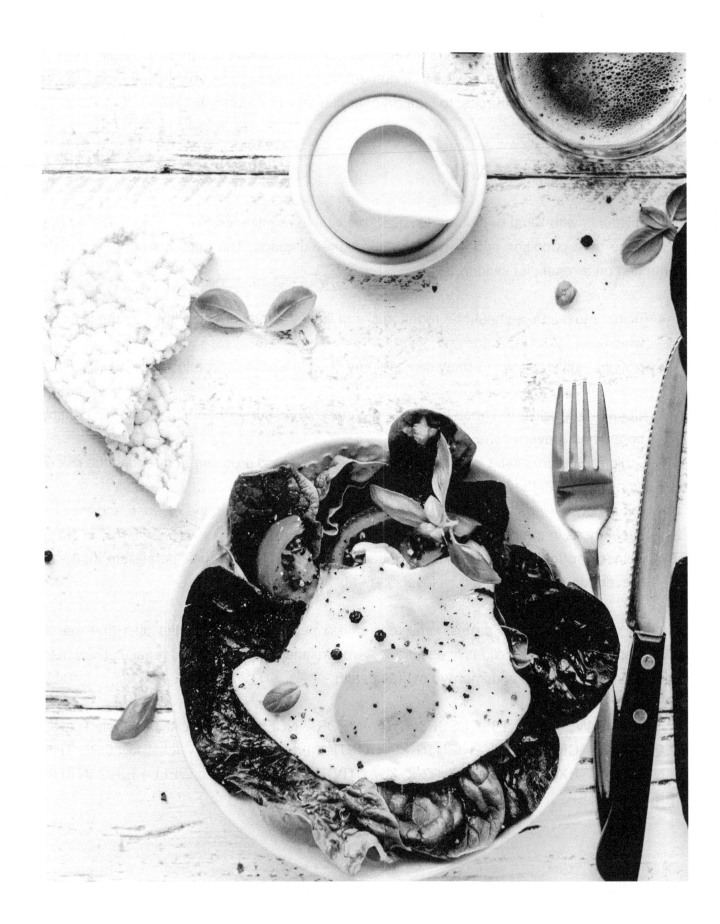

EXERCISE

Chapter 4

Benefits of Exercise

Types of Exercise

Exercise Guidelines

Incorporating Exercise into Daily Life

Overcoming Barriers to Exercise

Renal disease can be a wake-up call to better care for us and our bodies. Let us make every day count!

Regular exercise is essential for everyone, particularly for individuals with kidney disease. Exercise has numerous benefits for individuals with kidney disease, including improving cardiovascular health, reducing inflammation, and reducing stress and anxiety. Furthermore, exercise can help individuals with kidney disease manage their symptoms and slow the progression of the disease. Exercise can also help individuals with kidney disease maintain a healthy weight and improve their overall quality of life.

Despite the many benefits of exercise, many individuals with kidney disease may hesitate to start an exercise program. They may worry about overexerting themselves or exacerbating their symptoms. However, with proper guidance and a personalized exercise plan, individuals with kidney disease can safely and effectively incorporate exercise into their daily routines.

IN THIS CHAPTER, WE WILL DISCUSS THE BENEFITS OF EXERCISE FOR INDIVIDUALS WITH KIDNEY DISEASE, THE SUITABLE EXERCISE TYPES, AND GUIDELINES FOR EXERCISING SAFELY AND EFFECTIVELY. LET US GET STARTED!

BENEFITS OF EXERCISE

The kidneys are the body's filter, and just like any filter, they need to be cleaned and maintained regularly to function properly. Regular exercise has numerous mental and physical health benefits for those with kidney disease. These benefits include:

- IMPROVING CARDIOVASCULAR HEALTH: Kidney disease enhances the risk of heart disease, which can lead to strokes and heart attacks. Exercise can help improve heart health by strengthening the heart and blood vessels, reducing blood pressure, and improving cholesterol levels.
- IMPROVING BONE HEALTH: People with kidney disease risk developing the bone disease due to imbalances in minerals such as calcium and phosphorus. Exercises that place weight on the body, such as walking or lifting weights, can fortify bones and lower the chance of fractures.
- REDUCING INFLAMMATION: Inflammation is a widespread problem for individuals with kidney disease. It can contribute to various symptoms, such as fatigue and joint pain. Exercise has been shown to reduce inflammation, which can help alleviate these symptoms.
- REDUCING STRESS AND ANXIETY: Kidney disease can be stressful and anxiety-

inducing, particularly for individuals who require dialysis or a kidney transplant. Exercise can help reduce anxiety and stress by releasing endorphins. Endorphins are natural mood boosters.

- MANAGING SYMPTOMS AND SLOWING DISEASE PROGRESSION: Regular exercise can help manage symptoms such as fatigue and muscle weakness and can also slow the progression of renal disease by improving blood flow to the kidneys.

In addition to these benefits, exercise can help individuals with kidney disease maintain a healthy weight, improve their energy levels, and improve their overall quality of life.

However, it is vital to note that the benefits of exercise may vary depending on the individual's stage of kidney disease and overall health. It is essential to consult with a healthcare provider before starting an exercise program and to tailor the exercise plan to the individual's specific needs.

TYPES OF EXERCISE

Individuals with kidney disease can incorporate many distinct types of exercise into their daily routine, both at home and at a gym. Some examples include:

- BALANCE EXERCISES: Balance exercises, such as standing on one leg or using a balance board, can help improve stability and prevent falls. These exercises are essential for individuals with kidney disease who may experience dizziness or balance problems due to medication side effects.
- AEROBIC EXERCISE: Aerobic exercise, also known as cardio, is any exercise that increases heart and breathing rates. This type of exercise is beneficial for improving cardiovascular health and overall fitness. Aerobic exercise includes jogging, walking, swimming, cycling, and dancing.
- STRENGTH TRAINING: Strength training, also known as resistance training, involves using weights or resistance bands to build and maintain muscle mass. This type of exercise is essential for individuals with kidney disease, as they may experience muscle wasting or weakness. Examples of strength training exercises include using resistance bands, lifting weights, and doing bodyweight exercises such as push-ups or squats.
- FLEXIBILITY EXERCISES: Flexibility exercises, such as stretching or yoga, are essential for maintaining joint mobility and preventing injury. These exercises can also help improve balance and coordination. Examples of flexibility exercises include dynamic stretching, static stretching, yoga, and Pilates.

- LOW-IMPACT EXERCISE: Low-impact exercises, such as walking, cycling, or swimming, can benefit individuals with joint pain or other medical conditions that make high-impact exercise difficult. These exercises are also suitable for beginners or those just starting an exercise program.

It is essential to note that individuals with renal disease should consult with their healthcare provider before starting an exercise program. They may need to modify exercises or avoid certain activities based on their health status. Additionally, it is vital to start slowly and gradually increase the intensity and duration of your training over time. It will help you avoid injuries and improve your overall fitness.

EXERCISE GUIDELINES

When it comes to exercise, there are general guidelines that everyone should follow, as well as specific guidelines for individuals with kidney disease. The American Heart Association suggests at least 150 minutes of moderate-intensity aerobic exercise or 75 minutes of vigorous-intensity aerobic activity per week, spread out over at least three days. In addition to aerobic exercise, strength training exercises should be done at least two days per week. Including flexibility exercises as part of a well-rounded exercise program is also essential.

▶ EXERCISE GUIDELINES FOR INDIVIDUALS WITH KIDNEY DISEASE

Individuals with kidney disease may need to modify their exercise routine based on their health status. For example, those with advanced kidney disease may need to avoid high-impact exercises that could stress their joints. Additionally, individuals with kidney disease may need to be mindful of their fluid balance during training, as they may be on fluid restrictions.
Here are some general exercise guidelines for individuals with kidney disease:

- STAY HYDRATED: It is essential to drink enough fluids before, during, and after exercise to avoid dehydration. However, individuals on fluid restrictions should consult with their healthcare provider before increasing their fluid intake.
- START SLOWLY: If you are new to exercise or have not been physically active in a while, start slowly and gradually boost the intensity and duration of exercise over time.
- BE MINDFUL OF POTASSIUM: Some high-potassium foods, such as bananas and oranges, are commonly consumed during exercise. However, individuals with kidney disease may need to limit their intake of these foods.

- MONITOR YOUR BLOOD PRESSURE: Exercise can cause a temporary increase in blood pressure, so individuals with kidney disease should monitor their blood pressure before, during, and after exercise.
- CHOOSE LOW-IMPACT EXERCISES: Low-impact exercises, such as walking, cycling, or swimming, can be easier on the joints and are a good option for individuals with joint pain or other medical conditions that make high-impact exercise difficult.

By following these exercise guidelines, individuals with kidney disease can safely incorporate exercise into their daily routine to enjoy well-being.

INCORPORATING EXERCISE INTO DAILY LIFE

Incorporating exercise into daily life can be a challenge for anyone. Still, it can be especially difficult for individuals with kidney disease who may be dealing with symptoms such as fatigue and muscle weakness. However, regular exercise is vital for managing kidney disease and improving overall health. Here are some practical tips for incorporating exercise into daily life:

- SCHEDULE EXERCISE: By scheduling exercise at the same time each day, it will become part of your routine, making it easier to stick to. For example, you may exercise for 30 minutes after dinner each night.
- SET ACHIEVABLE GOALS: Setting achievable goals can help keep you motivated and give you a sense of accomplishment. Start with small goals, such as exercising for 10 minutes a day. Gradually increase the duration and intensity of your workouts.
- BE FLEXIBLE: Life can be unpredictable, and sometimes it is impossible to stick to a set exercise routine. If you miss a workout, do not beat yourself up. Instead, try to fit in some physical activity throughout the day. It can be about walking during your lunch break or taking the stairs instead of the elevator.
- MAKE IT ENJOYABLE: Exercise does not have to be a chore. Find activities you enjoy, such as dancing, swimming, or gardening. You are more likely to stick with an exercise routine if you want it.
- FIND A WORKOUT PARTNER: A workout partner can help keep you motivated and accountable. You can encourage each other and celebrate each other's progress. If you cannot find a workout partner, consider joining an online exercise group or forum.

Incorporating exercise into daily life can take effort, but the benefits are worth it. By following these tips, you can make exercise a regular part of your routine and improve your overall health.

OVERCOMING BARRIERS TO EXERCISE

Exercise is integral to managing kidney disease, but staying motivated and consistent with an exercise routine can be challenging. Some common barriers to exercise include more time, energy, and motivation. Fortunately, many strategies can help individuals overcome these barriers and stay on track with their exercise routine.

One of the most effective ways to overcome barriers to exercise is to set achievable goals. For example, if you are new to exercise, start with a small goal, such as walking for 10 minutes daily, and gradually increase your plan. You are finding an exercise you enjoy, whether walking, swimming, or dancing, is essential. When you want the activity, you are more likely to stick with it. Another strategy for overcoming barriers to exercise is to schedule training in your daily routine. Choose a time of day when you have the most energy and prioritize exercise. Consider finding a workout partner to help keep you accountable and motivated.

Fatigue can also be a common barrier to exercise, especially for individuals with kidney disease. If you are tired during the day, try breaking up your exercise into smaller sessions throughout the day. For example, you could do 10 minutes of activity in the morning, afternoon, and evening. Finally, it is essential to remember that exercise does not have to be perfect. It is okay to have off days or to modify your exercise routine based on how you feel that day. The key is to stay consistent and make exercise a regular part of your daily routine.

CHAPTER SUMMARY

Regular exercise can be a valuable tool in managing kidney disease. It offers many physical and mental health benefits, such as improving cardiovascular health, reducing inflammation, and reducing stress and anxiety. With various types of exercises available, individuals with kidney disease can choose what suits them best, such as aerobic exercise, strength training, and flexibility exercises.

Incorporating exercise into daily life can also be achieved by scheduling exercise at the same time each day, finding a workout partner, and setting achievable goals. Lastly, common barriers to exercise can be overcome by finding ways to make exercise enjoyable and rewarding. By making exercise a part of their daily routine, individuals with kidney disease can enjoy a healthier lifestyle and better manage their condition.

OUR KIDNEYS WORK HARD DAILY, SO LET US DO OUR PART TO SUPPORT
THEM. STAY HYDRATED, EAT A HEALTHY DIET, AND EXERCISE REGULARLY

* * * * * * * * * * *

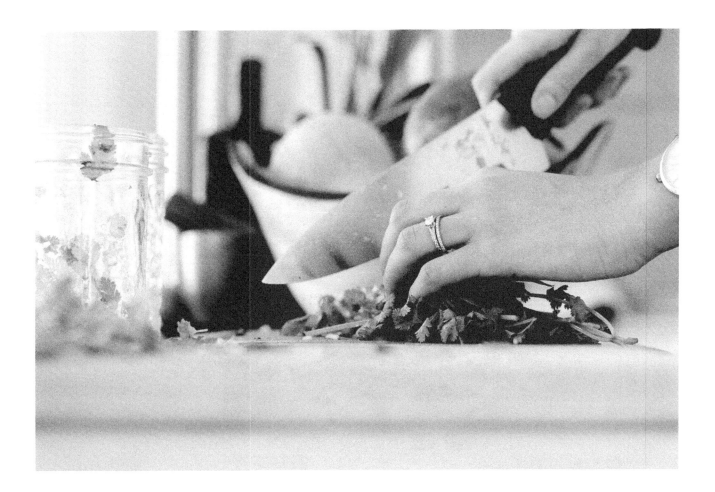

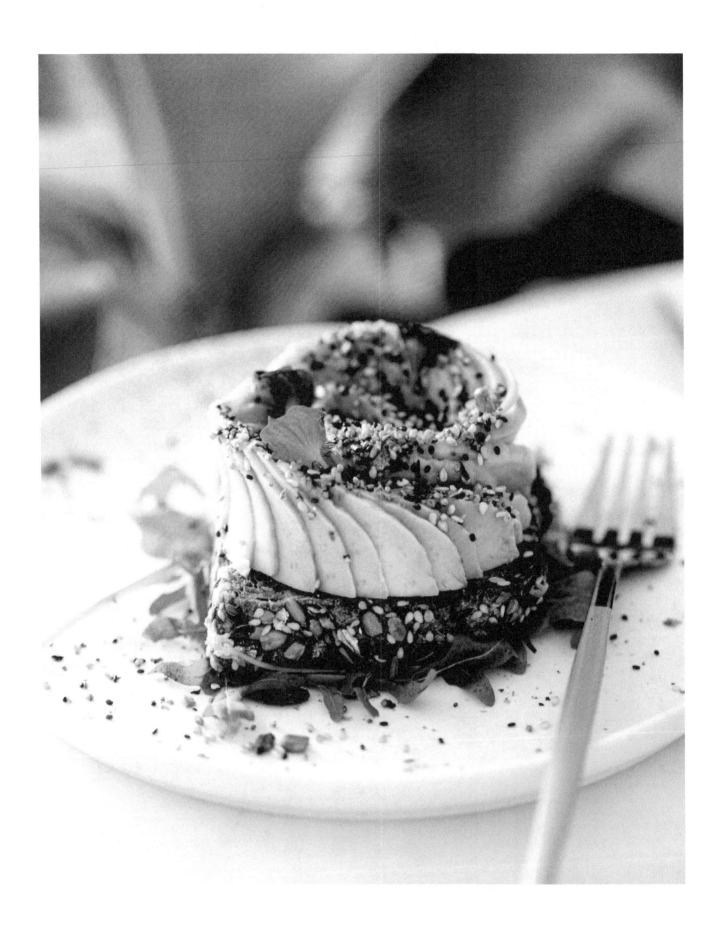

Chapter 5

FAQs

Benefits of Exercise

Types of Exercise

Exercise Guidelines

Incorporating Exercise into Daily Life

Overcoming Barriers to Exercise

CAN I USE MEAT SUBSTITUTES FOR PROTEIN SOURCES?

Yes, you can use meat substitutes as a protein source in a renal diet. However, choosing substitutes that are low in sodium and phosphorus is vital. Some good options include tofu, seitan, tempeh, and legumes such as beans, lentils, and chickpeas.

WHY IS ALCOHOL ON THE DO NOT LIST OF THE RENAL DIET?

Alcohol is on the do not list of the renal diet because it can be hard on the kidneys and cause dehydration. Alcohol can also interact with medications commonly used to treat kidney disease, making them less effective.

SHOULD I LOWER MY LIQUID INTAKE ON A RENAL DIET?

It depends on your situation. People with kidney disease may need to limit their fluid intake if they have excess fluid build up or are on dialysis. Your healthcare provider can provide specific guidance on fluid intake based on your medical history and current kidney function.

WHAT CAN I DO ABOUT MY LOW APPETITE?

Low appetite is a common issue for people with kidney disease. Some strategies to help increase appetite include eating smaller, more frequent meals throughout the day, incorporating high-calorie snacks such as nuts and seeds, and trying new foods and flavors to increase the enjoyment of meals.

WHAT ARE COMMON DIETARY RESTRICTIONS IN A RENAL DIET?

Common dietary restrictions in a renal diet include limiting sodium, potassium, and phosphorus intake and moderating protein intake. This may mean avoiding high-sodium processed foods, limiting high-potassium fruits and vegetables, and choosing lower-phosphorus protein sources such as lean meats, fish, and tofu.

IS IT SAFE TO CONSUME DAIRY PRODUCTS ON A RENAL DIET?

Dairy products are good protein, calcium, and other vital nutrients source. However, individuals with kidney disease may need to limit their intake of dairy products due to their phosphorus and potassium content. It is critical to discuss with a healthcare provider to determine how much dairy is appropriate for your individual needs.

CAN I STILL EAT WHOLE GRAINS ON A RENAL DIET?

Yes, whole grains can be included in a renal diet. However, it is crucial to be mindful of their phosphorus content and to choose lower phosphorus options such as brown rice, quinoa, and bulgur wheat. It is also essential to measure portion sizes and speak with a healthcare provider or registered dietitian to determine how much whole grains are appropriate for your needs.

WHAT ARE SOME RECOMMENDED SNACKS FOR A RENAL DIET?

Good snack options for a renal diet include fresh fruits, low-potassium vegetables, unsalted nuts and seeds, low-fat yogurt or cottage cheese, and air-popped popcorn. It is essential to be mindful of portion sizes and choose snacks low in sodium, phosphorus, and potassium.

HOW DOES A RENAL DIET AFFECT MY BLOOD PRESSURE?

A renal diet can help lower blood pressure, which is vital for individuals with kidney disease. The diet includes foods that are high in potassium and low in sodium, which can assist in lowering blood pressure. It is also essential to maintain a healthy weight, exercise regularly, and take medications as a healthcare provider prescribes.

CAN I EAT OUT AT RESTAURANTS WHILE ON A RENAL DIET?

Yes, eating out at restaurants while on a renal diet is possible. Review the menu beforehand and choose options lower in sodium, potassium, and phosphorus. Communicating any dietary restrictions to the server or chef is also essential.

ARE THERE ANY SUPPLEMENTS I SHOULD TAKE WHILE ON A RENAL DIET?

It is essential to talk to your healthcare provider before starting any supplements. Some supplements, such as iron or vitamin D, may be beneficial for people with kidney disease, but others may be harmful or interact with medications. Getting guidance from a healthcare provider before starting any supplements is essential.

HOW CAN I MANAGE MY POTASSIUM LEVELS ON A RENAL DIET?

Individuals with kidney disease may need to limit their potassium intake, which is found in many fruits and vegetables. Some tips for managing potassium levels include choosing low-potassium fruits and vegetables, such as apples and green beans, and cooking or soaking high-potassium foods before eating them.

CAN I STILL EAT SWEETS AND DESSERTS ON A RENAL DIET?

While sweets and desserts should be limited on a renal diet due to their sugar content, some options can still be enjoyed in moderation. Examples include sugar-free gelatin, low-fat frozen yogurt, and baked goods made with low-phosphorus ingredients. It is essential to be mindful of portion sizes and choose options that fit the diet's guidelines.

WHAT ARE SOME EASY MEAL IDEAS FOR A RENAL DIET?

Some easy meal ideas for a renal diet include grilled chicken with roasted vegetables, quinoa salad with cucumber and tomato, and baked salmon with brown rice and steamed broccoli. It is essential to measure portion sizes and choose foods low in phosphorus, sodium, and potassium.

HOW DOES A RENAL DIET AFFECT MY CHOLESTEROL LEVELS?

A renal diet can help lower cholesterol levels, which is vital for individuals with kidney disease. The diet includes foods low in cholesterol and saturated fat, such as low-fat dairy products and lean proteins. It is also essential to maintain a healthy weight, exercise regularly, and take medications as a healthcare provider prescribes.

* * * * * * * * * * * * * * * *

A RENAL DIET DOES NOT HAVE TO BE BORING. WITH SOME CREATIVITY, WE CAN CREATE DELICIOUS AND NUTRITIOUS MEALS THAT SUPPORT OUR KIDNEY HEALTH. DO NOT STOP NOW! THE STORY IS JUST GETTING STARTED. SO, LET US LOOK AT SOME FANTASTIC RECIPES IN THE FOLLOWING CHAPTERS.

* * * * * * * * * * * * * * * *

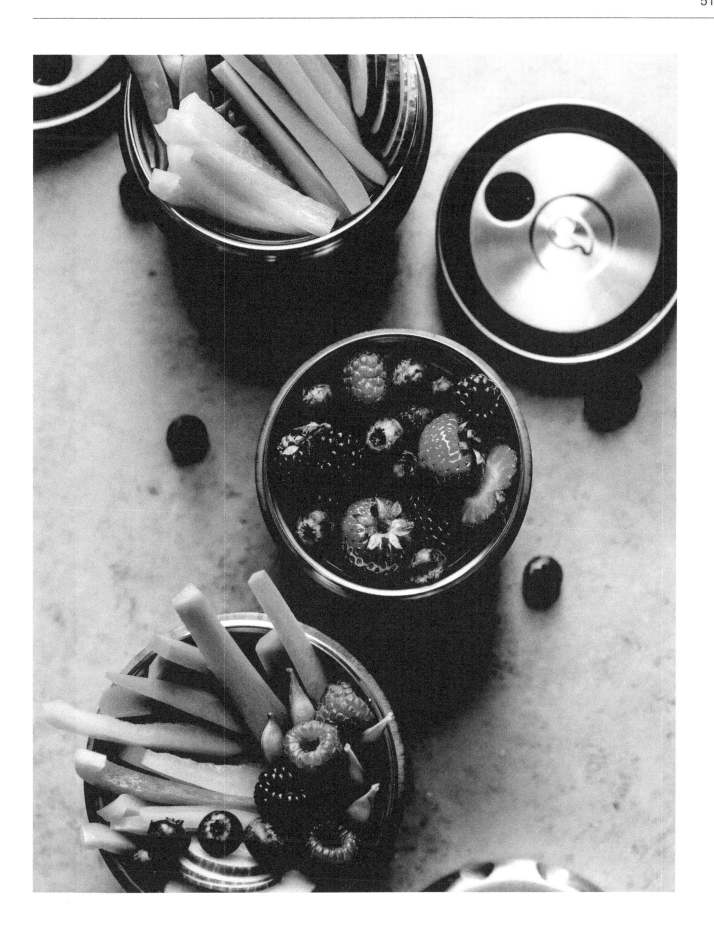

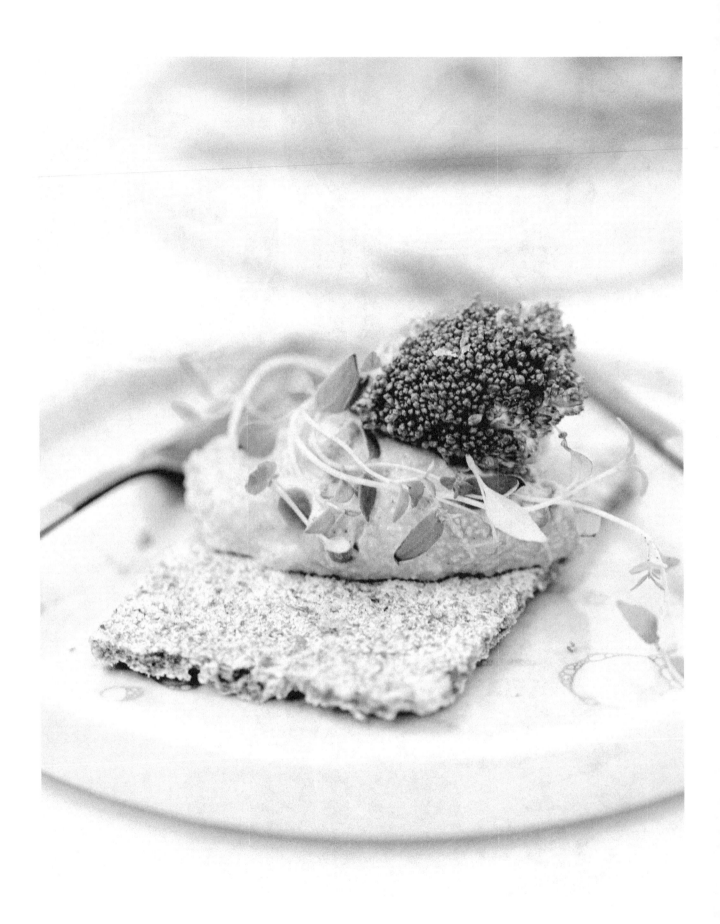

Chapter 6

BREAKFAST RECIPES

1. Coconut Breakfast Smoothie

2. Shrimp Bruschetta

3. Cheese Coconut Pancakes

4. Feta Mint Omelet

5. Turkey Burgers

6. Watermelon-Raspberry Smoothie

7. Mixed-Grain Hot Cereal

8. French Toast

9. Corn Pudding

10. Herbed Omelet

11. Egg and Veggie Muffins

12. Blueberry-Pineapple Smoothie

13. Festive Berry Parfait

14. Fruit and Oat Pancakes

15. Mexican Brunch Eggs

BREAKFAST IS THE MOST IMPORTANT MEAL OF THE DAY!

THIS CHAPTER OFFERS A VARIETY OF KIDNEY-FRIENDLY OPTIONS FOR BREAKFAST THAT ARE NOT ONLY HEALTHY BUT ALSO DELICIOUS. FROM COCONUT BREAKFAST SMOOTHIE TO MEXICAN BRUNCH EGGS, THESE RECIPES ARE EASY TO MAKE AND PERFECT FOR THOSE ON A RENAL DIET. START YOUR DAY OFF RIGHT WITH THESE SATISFYING BREAKFAST IDEAS

1. COCONUT BREAKFAST SMOOTHIE

Servings: 4   **Duration: 10 minutes**

INGREDIENTS	INSTRUCTIONS
• 2 cups coconut milk (low-fat) • 1 cup ice cubes • ½ cup fresh coconut chunks • 2 tbsp Keto maple syrup/ stevia or any sweetener of your choice	1. Add 2 cups of coconut milk, 2 tbsp of any sweetener, and ½ cup of coconut chunks to a high-speed blender and blend well until everything is mixed. 2. Now add ice cubes and blend for 1 minute until it becomes a thick consistency. ***Serve and enjoy your smoothie with berries on top(optional)***.

NUTRIENTS (PER SERVING):
Calories: 70 | Protein: 1g | Carbs: 5g | Fat: 6g | Sodium: 5mg | Potassium: 36mg | Fiber: 1g

2. SHRIMP BRUSCHETTA

Servings: 6   **Duration: 25 minutes**

INGREDIENTS	INSTRUCTIONS
• 4 tomatoes, ripe, diced • ½ cup olive oil • 1 tbsp lemon juice • 8 oz shrimp, cooked, small • ¼ tsp garlic powder • 1 tbsp fresh basil, chopped • 4 tbsp balsamic vinegar • 1 Italian loaf bread • ¼ tsp black pepper	1. Heat the oven and broil. Rinse the shrimp and set it in a colander to drain. Put the diced tomatoes, ¼ tsp garlic powder, ¼ tsp black pepper, ½ cup olive oil, 1 tbsp basil, 4 tbsp balsamic vinegar and 1 tbsp lemon juice in a bowl and mix together. 2. Spread olive oil on 1/4-inch-thick slices of bread, place under the broiler, and toast for 5 minutes or until lightly brown. Remove from oven. 3. Place the shrimp mixture on the toast. Serve immediately.

NUTRIENTS (PER SERVING):
Protein: 8g | Carbs: 9g | Fat: 3g | Iron: 0.6mg

3. CHEESE COCONUT PANCAKES

Servings: 4   **Duration: 20 minutes**

INGREDIENTS	INSTRUCTIONS
• 4 eggs • 1/2 cup coconut Flour • 1 cup cottage cheese • 2 tbsp coconut oil • ½ tsp baking powder • 1 tsp vanilla Extract • 1/2 tsp salt	1. Put 1 cup of cottage cheese and 4 eggs in a blender. 2. Blend until everything is mixed well. 3. Pour the ingredients from the blender into a bowl and add half cup of coconut flour, ½ teaspoon of salt, ½ tsp of baking soda, and 1 tsp of vanilla extract. Mix it well, then let it sit for 5 minutes. As the mixture sits, it will get thicker. 4. Put 2 tbsp or more of Coconut Oil into a frying pan and reduce the heat to low. Put ¼ cup of batter on the frying pan. 5. Cook for approximately 3 minutes on one side and 2 minutes after turning. 6. Serve the pancakes on a platter and top them with your favorite fresh fruits or sugar-free syrup. Enjoy your Cheese Coconut Pancakes!

NUTRIENTS (PER SERVING):
Protein: 14.4g | Carbs: 10.4g | Fat: 17.0g

4. FETA MINT OMELET

Servings: 1   **Duration: 15 minutes**

INGREDIENTS	INSTRUCTIONS
• 3 eggs • 2 tbsp crumbled feta • A handful of fresh chopped mint • 2 tbsp milk • ½ tsp olive oil • Pinch of salt & pepper	1. In a bowl, beat the eggs with all the other ingredients except the olive oil. 2. Take a heavy, medium-sized pan, and heat the olive oil on low flame. 3. Add the egg mixture, making sure it covers the whole pan evenly. 4. Let it cook until the bottoms are firmed, but the top is still liquid. 5. Fold in half carefully using a rubber spatula. 6. *Sprinkle feta cheese on top, cut into slices and serve.*

NUTRIENTS (PER SERVING):
Carbs: 4g | Protein: 9g | Sugar: 1.6g | Fat: 3.3g | Fiber: 11g

5. TURKEY BURGERS

Servings: 2   **Duration: 15 minutes**

INGREDIENTS

- ¼ tsp garlic powder (not garlic salt)
- 1 tsp parsley flakes
- 1 lb. lean organic ground turkey
- ½ tsp onion powder (not onion salt
- 1 tbsp liquid smoke
- 1 lb. lean organic ground turkey
- ½ tsp fresh ground pepper

INSTRUCTIONS

1. Preheat the grill for at least 5 minutes to get it hot.
2. Mix the onion powder, ground turkey, pepper, garlic powder, parsley, and liquid smoke well in a bowl. Form into 4 oz patties.
3. Put on the grill and shut the lid. For 4–6 minutes, grill. Serve on a bun with less sodium and with traditional burger toppings.

NUTRIENTS (PER SERVING):

Calories: 269 | Carbs: 4g | Protein: 11g | Fat: 13g | Sugar: 1g

6. WATERMELON-RASPBERRY SMOOTHIE

Servings: 2   **Duration: 10 minutes**

INGREDIENTS

- 1 cup ice
- ½ cup fresh raspberries
- ½ cup boiled, cooled, and shredded red cabbage
- 1 cup diced watermelon

INSTRUCTIONS

1. Put the cabbage in the blender and pulse it for 2 minutes or until it is finely chopped.
2. Add the watermelon and raspberries, pulse for about a minute.
3. Add ice and blend the smoothie until it is very smooth and thick. Put the liquid in two glasses. ***Let the smoothie be completely chilled and serve with raspberry (optional) on top.***

NUTRIENTS (PER SERVING):

Calories: 47 | Fat: 0g | Carbs: 11g | Phosphorus: 30mg | Potassium: 197mg | Sodium: 4mg | Protein: 1g

7. MIXED-GRAIN HOT CEREAL

Servings: 4 **Duration: 10 minutes**

INGREDIENTS	INSTRUCTIONS
• 2¼ cups water • 6 tbsp uncooked bulgur • 6 tbsp plain uncooked couscous • 2 tbsp uncooked whole buckwheat • 1¼ cups vanilla rice milk • 1 cup peeled, sliced apple • ½ tsp. ground cinnamon	1. In a medium-sized saucepan, heat the water and milk over medium-high heat. 2. Bring it to a boil, then add apple, bulgur, and buckwheat. Reduce the heat to low and let the bulgur cook, stirring occasionally, for 20 to 25 minutes or until soft. 3. Remove the saucepan from the heat and combine the couscous and cinnamon with the liquid. Cover the saucepan and let it sit for 10 minutes. Finally, use a fork to fluff the cereal before serving.

NUTRIENTS (PER SERVING):
Calories: 159 | Carbs: 34g | Phosphorus: 130mg | Fat: 1g | Potassium: 116mg | Sodium: 33mg | Protein: 4g

8. FRENCH TOAST

Servings: 4 **Duration: 15 minutes**

INGREDIENTS	INSTRUCTIONS
• ¼ cup 1% milk • ¼ tsp allspice • 4 large egg whites, slightly beaten • 4 slices white bread • ½ tsp cinnamon • 1 tbsp margarine	1. Mix egg whites with milk, cinnamon, and allspice. 2. Dip one piece of bread at a time into the batter. 3. Place on a hot grill or in a skillet with melted margarine. 4. When the bread is golden brown, turn it. ***Serve warm with maple syrup drizzle on top (sugar-free if diabetic)***.

NUTRIENTS (PER SERVING):
Calories: 125 | Protein: 7g | Cholesterol: 0mg | Potassium: 128mg | Fat: 4g | Carbs: 14g | Phosphorus: 61mg

9. CORN PUDDING

Servings: 6   **Duration: 40 minutes**

INGREDIENTS	INSTRUCTIONS
• 1 tbsp. unsalted butter for greasing the baking dish	1. Preheat the oven to 350°F.
• 3 eggs	2. Butter a baking dish 8 inches by 8 inches and set it aside.
• ¾ cup unsweetened rice milk, at room temperature	3. Add the baking soda and flour substitute to a small bowl and set it aside.
• 2 tbsp granulated sugar	4. Mix the rice milk, eggs, butter, sour cream, and sugar in a medium bowl.
• 2 tbsp all-purpose flour	5. Mix the flour mixture into the egg mixture until it is smooth.
• 2 cups frozen corn kernels, thawed	6. Stir the corn into the batter until it is well blended.
• 3 tbsp unsalted butter, melted	7. Put the batter in the baking dish and bake for about 40 minutes or until the pudding is set.
• ½ tsp Ener-G baking soda substitute	8. Let the pudding cool for about 15 minutes and serve.
• 2 tbsp light sour cream	

NUTRIENTS (PER SERVING):
Calories: 175 | Fat: 10g | Carbs: 19g | Phosphorus: 111mg | Potassium: 170mg | Sodium: 62mg | Protein: 5g

10. HERBED OMELET

Servings: 2   **Duration: 15 minutes**

INGREDIENTS	INSTRUCTIONS
• 1 ½ tsp vegetable oil	1. Beat eggs, and add water & spices. Set aside.
• ⅛ tsp tarragon	2. Over medium heat, heat the oil in an 8-inch frying pan. Add the onions and sauté. Take out of the pan.
• ¼ tsp parsley (optional)	3. Pour the mixture into a hot frying pan over medium heat.
• 2 tbsp water	4. As the omelet cooks, lift it with a spoon to let the uncooked part flow to the bottom.
• 1 tbsp chopped onion	5. ***When the omelet is done, transfer it to a serving platter and top it with the crispy cooked onion. (optional)***. Enjoy and serve immediately!
• 4 eggs	
• ¼ tsp basil	

NUTRIENTS (PER SERVING):
Calories: 159 | Protein: 14g | Cholesterol: 474mg | Potassium: 157mg | Carbs: 0g | Phosphorus: 214mg | Fiber: 0g | Calcium: 60mg

11. EGG AND VEGGIE MUFFINS

Servings: 4 **Duration: 20 minutes**

INGREDIENTS	INSTRUCTIONS
• 4 eggs • 2 tbsp. unsweetened rice milk • ½ red bell pepper, finely chopped • Cooking spray, for greasing the muffin pans • ½ sweet onion, finely chopped • Pinch freshly ground black pepper • 1 tbsp chopped fresh parsley • Pinch red pepper flakes	1. Set the oven temperature to 350° F. 2. Spray 4 muffin pans with cooking spray and set it aside. 3. Whisk the eggs, milk, onion, red pepper, parsley, red pepper flakes, and black pepper together in a large bowl until everything is mixed. 4. Pour the egg mixture into the muffin tins that have been set up. 5. Bake the muffins for 18 to 20 minutes until golden and puffed. Serve hot or cold.

NUTRIENTS (PER SERVING):
Calories: 84 | Fat: 5g | Carbs: 3g | Phosphorus: 110mg | Potassium: 117mg | Sodium: 75mg | Protein: 7g

12. BLUEBERRY-PINEAPPLE SMOOTHIE

Servings: 2 **Duration: 15 minutes**

INGREDIENTS	INSTRUCTIONS
• ½ cup water • ½ cup pineapple chunks • ½ cup English cucumber • 1 cup frozen blueberries • ½ apple	1. Put the apple, pineapple, blueberries, cucumber, and water in a blender until the mixture is thick and smooth. 2. Put the liquid in two glasses and serve. ***Top with the leftover blueberries and mint leaf (optional). Enjoy!***

NUTRIENTS (PER SERVING):
Calories: 87 | Fat: 1g | Carbs: 22g | Phosphorus: 28mg | Potassium: 192mg | Sodium: 3mg | Protein: 1g

13. FESTIVE BERRY PARFAIT

Servings: 4 **Duration: 20 minutes (+1 hour to chill)**

INGREDIENTS	INSTRUCTIONS
• 1 cup crumbled Meringue Cookies • ½ tsp ground cinnamon • 1 tbsp granulated sugar • 1 cup vanilla rice milk, at room temperature • 2 cups fresh blueberries • ½ cup plain cream cheese, at room temperature • 1 cup sliced fresh strawberries	1. Whisk the milk, sugar, cream cheese and cinnamon together in a small bowl until smooth. 2. Pour a quarter cup of cookie crumbs into the bottom of each of the 4 6-ounce glasses. 3. Spread 1/4 cup of the mixture with cream cheese on top of the cookies. 4. Put a quarter cup of the berries on top of the cream cheese. 5. Repeat with the cookies, the cream cheese mixture, and the berries in each cup. 6. Put in the fridge for 1 hour to chill and serve.

NUTRIENTS (PER SERVING):

Fat: 11g | Carbs: 25g | Phosphorus: 84mg | Potassium: 189mg | Sodium: 145mg | Protein: 4g

14. FRUIT AND OAT PANCAKES

Servings: 4 **Duration: 20 minutes**

INGREDIENTS	INSTRUCTIONS
• 1/2 cup rolled oats • 1 egg • 1 tbsp margarine • 1 cup flour • 1/2 tsp baking powder • 1 8-oz. can fruit cocktail, undrained • 1/2 cup liquid non-dairy creamer	1. In a bowl, mix together everything except margarine. 2. Melt margarine in a large skillet. 3. Pour about 1/4 cup of batter per pancake into the pan and cook over medium heat until the pancakes are bubbly in the middle and dry around the edges. 4. Flip pancakes with a spatula and cook until the bottoms are golden brown. **Serve it with a latte (optional) or any drink of your choice.**

NUTRIENTS (PER SERVING):

Carbs: 9g | Protein: 7g | Fat: 8g | Sodium: 152mg

15. MEXICAN BRUNCH EGGS

Servings: 8   **Duration: 20 minutes**

INGREDIENTS

- 8 eggs, beaten
- 2 tbsp margarine
- 2 tbsp chopped pimiento
- 1 ½ tsp ground cumin
- 2 cloves garlic, crushed
- 1/8 tsp cayenne pepper
- 2 cups unsalted corn chips
- 1 ½ cups frozen corn, thawed
- ½ cup chopped onion

INSTRUCTIONS

1. In a large skillet, melt the margarine and cook the garlic and onion until the onion is soft. Mix in the cayenne, cumin and corn. Stir to mix.
2. Pour in the eggs and cook, stirring occasionally, over low heat until the eggs are set.
3. Set corn chips out on a big plate. Put egg mixture on chips, and then sprinkle pimiento on top. Serve right away

NUTRIENTS (PER SERVING):

Calories: 214 | Carbs: 13g | Protein: 9g | Fat: 14g | Sodium: 147mg |
Potassium: 240mg | Phosphorus: 91mg

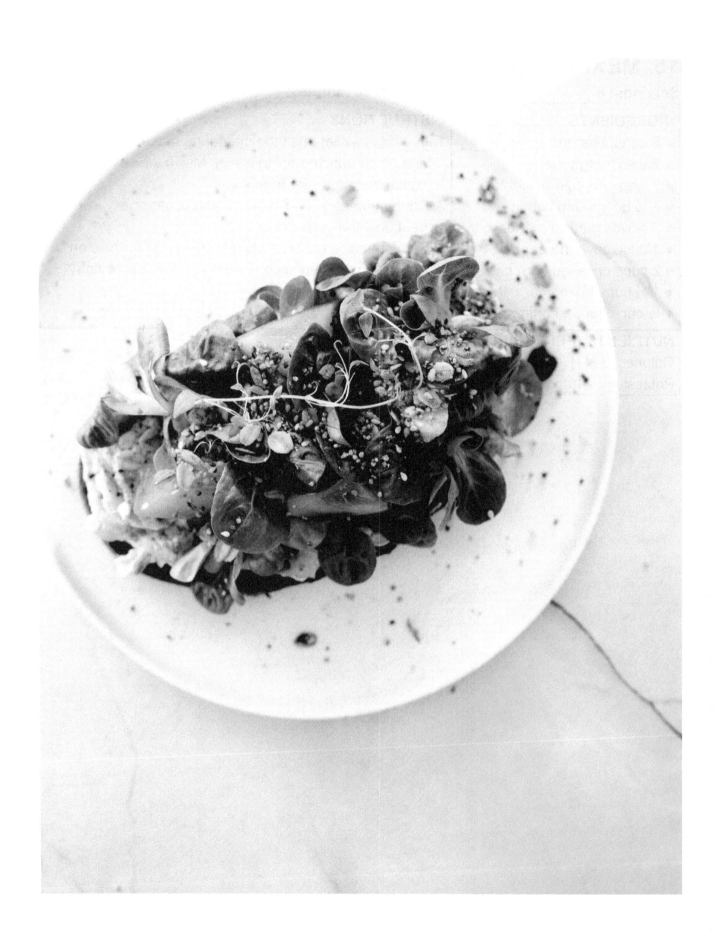

GRAINS, BEANS AND LEGUMES

Chapter 7

1. Vegetables Fried Rice

2. Colorful Bean Salad

3. Seasoned Green Beans

4. Vegetarian Egg Fried Rice

5. Rice O'Brien

6. Steamed Asparagus

7. Favorite Green Beans

8. New Orleans-Style Red Beans and Rice

9. Moroccan Couscous

10. Easy Lentil Soup

11. Summer Chickpea Salad

12. Stewed Pigeon Peas

13. Instant Pot Cilantro Lime Rice

14. Easy Popcorn Munch

15. Creamy Corn Soup

BEANS, BEANS, THEY ARE GOOD FOR YOUR HEART.
THE MORE YOU EAT, THE MORE YOU.

IN THIS CHAPTER, YOU WILL FIND A VARIETY OF RECIPES THAT INCORPORATE THESE NUTRIENT-DENSE FOODS INTO YOUR RENAL DIET. FROM VEGETABLES FRIED RICE TO MOROCCAN COUSCOUS, THESE RECIPES ARE BOTH DELICIOUS AND KIDNEY FRIENDLY. DISCOVER NEW WAYS TO INCORPORATE HEALTHY GRAINS, BEANS, AND LEGUMES INTO YOUR MEALS WITH THESE EASY-TO-FOLLOW RECIPES.

1. VEGETABLES FRIED RICE

Servings: 6   **Duration: 20 minutes**

INGREDIENTS	INSTRUCTIONS
• ½ cup peas • 1 tbsp olive oil • 1 tbsp grated fresh ginger • 1 cup sliced carrots • 2 tsp minced garlic • ½ cup green beans, cut into 1-inch pieces • ½ cup chopped eggplant • ½ sweet onion, chopped • 3 cups cooked rice • 2 tbsp chopped fresh cilantro	1. Heat the olive oil in a large pan over medium-high heat. 2. Sauté the onion, 1 tbsp grated ginger, and 2 tsp minced garlic for about 3 minutes or until softened. 3. Add eggplant, peas, carrots, and green beans, stir and cook for another 3 minutes. 4. Stir in rice and cilantro. 5. Stir constantly for about 10 minutes or until the rice is heated through. ***Serve with Indian curry or any combination dish. Enjoy!***

NUTRIENTS (PER SERVING):

Calories: 189 | Protein: 6g | Fat: 7g | Carbs: 28g | Phosphorus: 89mg | Potassium: 172mg | Sodium: 13mg

2. COLORFUL BEAN SALAD

Servings: 4 **Duration: 30 minutes**

INGREDIENTS

(For salad)
- 1 medium tomato, 3/8 inch dice
- 2 small scallions, in 3/8 inch slices
- 1 jalapeno, deseeded, minced (to taste)
- 1 yellow bell pepper, in 3/8 inch dice
- 2 tbsp basil, minced
- 2 (14-ounce) cans of kidney beans, rinsed and drained

(For dressing)
- 1/2 tsp sugar (to taste) or any sweetener
- 2 tbsp olive oil
- 2 ½ tbsp apple cider vinegar
- Pinch of salt & pepper
- 1 tsp Dijon mustard

INSTRUCTIONS
1. For the dressing, mix all ingredients, except for the oil, until everything is well combined. Taste and add oil. It should be perfectly sour.
2. Mix the salad ingredients in a large bowl, then pour the dressing on top and stir well.
3. Let the flavors combine for 15 minutes or keep in the refrigerator for up to one hour.

(Note)
If you want to make the salad ahead of time, do not add the basil until 30 minutes before serving. This way, the basil will not turn brown, and the flavors will have time to blend.

NUTRIENTS (PER SERVING):
Sodium: 644mg | Carbs: 8g | Fiber: 11.5g | Sugars: 5.3g | Protein: 11.3g | Cholesterol: 0mg

3. SEASONED GREEN BEANS

Servings: 4 **Duration: 5 minutes**

INGREDIENTS
- ½ tsp onion salt
- ¾ pound fresh green beans, trimmed
- ½ tsp garlic powder
- Freshly ground pepper to taste
- ½ tsp garlic salt
- 1 ½ tbsp olive oil

INSTRUCTIONS
1. Heat olive oil in a pan over medium heat.
2. Add onion salt, green beans, garlic powder, garlic salt, and black pepper to the pan.
3. Cook and stir continuously for 5 to 10 minutes or until the food is as soft as desired. Serve hot and enjoy!

NUTRIENTS (PER SERVING):
Calories: 74 | Carbs: 7g | Protein: 2g | Fat: 5g

4. VEGETARIAN EGG FRIED RICE

Servings: 6   **Duration: 40 minutes**

INGREDIENTS
- 4 cups rice, cooked
- 2 garlic cloves
- 3 tbsp canola oil
- ½ cup green peas
- 1 tbsp fresh ginger
- 1 cup yellow onion
- 1 tbsp reduced-sodium soy sauce
- 1 cup extra-firm tofu
- 2 medium carrots
- 2 green onions
- 6 large eggs
- ½ cup cilantro
- ¼ tsp dry mustard

INSTRUCTIONS
1. Mince the garlic and ginger root. Slice the carrots. Dice yellow onion and tofu. Chop cilantro and green onions.
2. Beat the six eggs, then cook in a skillet like an omelet. Chop cooked eggs into pieces and set aside.
3. Heat the oil in a skillet over medium heat. Stir in the garlic, ginger, carrots, yellow onion, tofu, peas, and dry mustard.
4. Add rice, soy sauce and chopped eggs when the carrots are softened. Mix for 2-3 minutes and remove heat.
5. Top with cilantro and green onions and serve hot.

NUTRIENTS (PER SERVING):
Calories: 342 | Carbs: 37g | Fat: 15g | Cholesterol: 212mg | Sodium: 238mg | Potassium: 350mg | Phosphorus: 230mg | Fiber: 3.2g | Protein: 15g

5. RICE O'BRIEN

Servings: 4   **Duration: 30 minutes**

INGREDIENTS
- 1½ cup water
- ½ cup onion, thinly sliced
- ½ tsp thyme
- ¼ cup carrots, shredded
- 1 tbsp lemon juice
- 1 cup rice, uncooked
- ½ tsp black pepper
- ¼ cup green pepper, chopped
- 1 tsp margarine
- ¼ tsp red pepper

INSTRUCTIONS
1. Put a large skillet over medium heat. Add margarine, chopped carrots, red pepper, green pepper, thyme, black pepper, Lemon juice, onion, and 1 ½ cup of water.
2. Let the mixture simmer for 5 to 6 minutes until all spices and vegetables are well combined.
3. Now add rice and let it simmer for another 6 to 7 minutes. Cover with a lid and cook on low heat for about 15 minutes. When done, fluff rice lightly with a fork. ***Serve hot and top with your favorite gravy. Enjoy healthy eating!***

NUTRIENTS (PER SERVING):
Calories: 207 | Protein: 4g | Potassium: 125mg | Fat: 3g | Carbs: 29g | Phosphorus: 46mg | Fiber: 1g

6. STEAMED ASPARAGUS

Servings: 3   **Duration: 20 minutes**

INGREDIENTS	INSTRUCTIONS
• 2 cups water • 1 tbsp lemon juice • 12 fresh asparagus spears • 2 tbsp margarine, melted (unsalted)	1. In a small bowl, combine the margarine and lemon juice, and set aside. 2. Fill the bottom of a steamer with water and bring it to a boil. 3. Place the asparagus on a steamer rack and position it over the boiling water. 4. Steam the asparagus until it turns bright green, which usually takes around 2 minutes. Check to see if it needs more time. 5. Once the asparagus is cooked to your desired tenderness, remove it from the steamer and transfer it to a serving plate. 6. Drizzle the lemon and margarine mixture over the asparagus and serve immediately. ***Enjoy your delicious and healthy steamed asparagus!***

NUTRIENTS (PER SERVING):

Calories: 62 | Trans Fat: 0g | Sodium: 1mg | Protein: 1g | Cholesterol: 0mg | Potassium: 123mg | Carbs: 3g | Fiber: 1g | Phosphorus: 32mg

7. FAVORITE GREEN BEANS

Servings: 6   **Duration: 40 minutes**

INGREDIENTS	INSTRUCTIONS
• 1 ½ cups unsalted top cracker crumbs • ½ cup fresh mushrooms, sliced • 1 tsp paprika • 1 small onion, chopped • 2 cans whole green beans, drained and rinsed • ¼ tsp coarse black pepper • 4 tbsp margarine, unsalted	1. Preheat the oven to 350°F. 2. In a large bowl, combine the green beans, chopped onion, sliced mushrooms, paprika, and black pepper. 3. Spread the mixture evenly into a greased baking dish. 4. Sprinkle the cracker crumbs over the top of the green bean casserole, then dot with margarine. 5. Bake for 30-35 minutes, or until the cracker crumbs are golden brown and the casserole is heated through. Serve warm and enjoy!

NUTRIENTS (PER SERVING):

Calories: 137 | Sodium: 77mg | Protein: 2g | Cholesterol: 0mg | Potassium: 214mg | Carbs: 14g | Phosphorus: 38mg | Fiber: 2g | Calcium: 38mg

8. NEW ORLEANS-STYLE RED BEANS AND RICE

Servings: 6   **Duration: 1 hour**

INGREDIENTS	INSTRUCTIONS
• 1 pound dried beans, sorted and rinsed • 2 ham hocks • 1 tsp seasoned salt • 2 tablespoons vegetable oil • 1 onion, chopped • 1 teaspoon dried thyme • 1 bay leaf • 1/4 teaspoon black pepper • Cooked rice, for serving	1. Rinse the dried beans and remove any debris or damaged beans. Place them in a large Dutch oven and add enough water to cover them by 2 inches. Bring the water to a boil and let the beans cook for 2 minutes. 2. Remove the Dutch oven from the heat, cover it with a lid, and let it sit for 1 hour. Drain the beans and set them aside. 3. Sprinkle 1/2 teaspoon of seasoned salt on each side of the ham hocks. 4. In the same Dutch oven, heat 2 tablespoons of vegetable oil over medium-high heat. Add the ham hocks and brown them for about 3 minutes on each side. 5. Stir in the reserved beans, chopped onion, thyme, bay leaf, 1/2 teaspoon of seasoned salt, and 4 cups of water. Bring the mixture to a boil. 6. Reduce the heat to low, cover the Dutch oven, and let the beans simmer for 45 minutes or until they are tender. Discard the bay leaf. 7. Serve the beans over cooked rice.

NUTRIENTS (PER SERVING):
Protein: 15g | Carbs: 24g | Fat: 15g | Cholesterol: 212mg | Sodium: 238mg | Potassium: 350mg | Phosphorus: 230mg | Fiber: 2g

9. MOROCCAN COUSCOUS

Servings: 4   **Duration: 10-15 minutes**

INGREDIENTS	INSTRUCTIONS
• 1 cup water • 2/3 cup dry couscous • ½ tbsp margarine or olive oil • 2 tbsp chopped onion	1. In the butter or olive oil, cook the chopped onion until it is soft. In a medium saucepan, bring water to a boil. 2. Add the couscous and onion and stir. Cook for 5 minutes with a lid on top. 3. Turn the stove off and let it sit for 5 minutes. Use a fork to lightly fluff the rice before serving.

NUTRIENTS (PER SERVING):
Calories:115 | Carbs: 21g | Protein: 3.5g | Fat: 2g | Sodium: 24mg | Potassium: 61mg

10. EASY LENTIL SOUP

Servings: 4   **Duration: 20 minutes**

INGREDIENTS	INSTRUCTIONS
• 6 cups (1 liter) vegetable stock/broth • 1 large onion, chopped • 6 medium carrots coarsely grated • 1.5 tbsp olive oil • 0.75 cup (100ml) milk dairy free • 1/13 cup (140g) dried red lentils uncooked • 1 ½ tsp ground cumin	1. In a large pot, heat the oil over medium heat. Add onion and cook it for 3 minutes until it becomes soft. 2. Mix in the carrots, lentils, stock, milk, and cumin, and bring to a boil. 3. Lower the heat and let the lentils cook for about 15 minutes. 4. Use a hand blender or food processor to make a puree. If you want to make it thin, add more water. ***Pour the soup into bowls and, if you want, add chopped fresh parsley and a mixture of seeds.***

NUTRIENTS (PER SERVING):

Calories: 218 | Carbs: 30g | Sugar: 6g | Protein: 11g | Fat: 4g | Vitamin C: 10mg | Potassium: 686mg | Fiber: 14g | Calcium: 92mg | Iron: 3.6mg | Sodium: 70mg

11. SUMMER CHICKPEA SALAD

Servings: 2   **Duration: 10 minutes**

INGREDIENTS	INSTRUCTIONS
• 2 oz. feta, crumbled • 1 tbsp extra-virgin olive oil • 2 small tomatoes, sliced • 1/4 tsp kosher salt • 15 oz. can chickpeas, rinsed and drained • ¼ cup red onion • 1 tsp lemon juice • 2 mini cucumbers, chopped • 1/8 tsp dried oregano	1. In a large bowl, toss the chickpeas, cucumbers, tomatoes, and red onion with ½ tsp lemon, ½ tbsp of olive oil, and salt. 2. Put half the material on each plate and top with feta, dried oregano, lemon juice and remaining olive oil.

NUTRIENTS (PER SERVING):

Carbs: 21g | Protein: 11g | Fat: 9g | Fiber: 11.5g

12. STEWED PIGEON PEAS

Servings: 4   **Duration: 25 minutes**

INGREDIENTS	INSTRUCTIONS
• ½ tbsp sazon seasoning, 1 packet • 1 tbsp olive oil • 15-ounce can of gandules, pigeon peas not drained • ¼ cup sofrito • ½ cup canned tomato sauce, half 8 oz. can • ½ tsp chicken or veggie bouillon • ½ cup water • cooked, long-grain white rice for serving(optional)	1. In a medium skillet, heat the olive oil and add the sofrito. Stir for 3 to 4 minutes while cooking. 2. Add the rest of the ingredients, bring to a boil, cover and let it simmer for 20 minutes until the flavors blend and the sauce thickens. 3. If you want the beans thicker, remove the lid and let simmer until thickened. To make the beans soupier, add more water. 4. Serve over white rice.

NUTRIENTS (PER SERVING):
Calories: 131 | Protein: 5g | Fiber: 4g | Fat: 4.5g | Carbs: 17.5g

13. INSTANT POT CILANTRO LIME RICE

Servings: 4   **Duration: 20 minutes**

INGREDIENTS	INSTRUCTIONS
• 1¼ cups water • 1 cup long-grain white rice or jasmine, un-rinsed • ½ lime cut into pieces • 2 tsp olive oil • 1/4 cup fresh chopped cilantro • ½ tsp kosher salt	1. Stir the rice, water, 1 tsp of oil, and salt in the pressure cooker pot. 2. Cover and cook for 3 minutes under high pressure. When the timer ends, let the pressure release naturally for 10 minutes. 3. After 10 minutes, do a quick pressure release and use a fork to fluff the rice. 4. Mix the chopped cilantro, lemon pieces, and the rest of the oil in a medium bowl. Add in rice and toss until well mixed. **_Serve on your desired platter and enjoy._**

NUTRIENTS (PER SERVING):
Calories: 194 | Carbs: 19g | Protein: 3g | Fat: 3.5g | Sodium: 280mg | Sugar: 0.5g

14. EASY POPCORN MUNCH

Servings: 8   **Duration: 7-8 minutes**

INGREDIENTS	INSTRUCTIONS
• 2 cups sweetened wheat puff cereal • 2 cups graham cracker cereal • 8 cups popped popcorn, unsalted • 1 stick unsalted butter • ½ Caramel syrup	1. In a microwavable bowl, combine cereals, butter, and popcorn. Pour caramel syrup over the top. Microwave for 1 ½ minutes on high or until hot. 2. Let it sit for 5 minutes. Break into pieces.

NUTRIENTS (PER SERVING):

Calories: 122 | Carbs: 20g | Protein: 2g | Fat: 4g | Sodium: 104mg | Potassium: 71mg | Phosphorus: 46mg

15. CREAMY CORN SOUP

Servings: 3   **Duration: 25 minutes**

INGREDIENTS	INSTRUCTIONS
• 1 cup liquid non-dairy creamer • 1 cup water • 2 tbsp flour • 1 ½ cups corn kernels, canned • 1/8 tsp pepper • 2 tbsp margarine • 2 jars (128g each) strained cream-style corn baby food	1. Melt the margarine in a saucepan over low heat. Add flour and pepper. Cook for 1 minute smooth. Stir in corn. 2. Slowly add non-dairy creamer and water. Cook until bubbles form. ***Serve warm.***

NUTRIENTS (PER SERVING):

Calories: 245 | Carbs: 22g | Protein: 3g | Fat: 16g | Sodium: 64mg | Potassium: 238mg | Phosphorus: 85mg

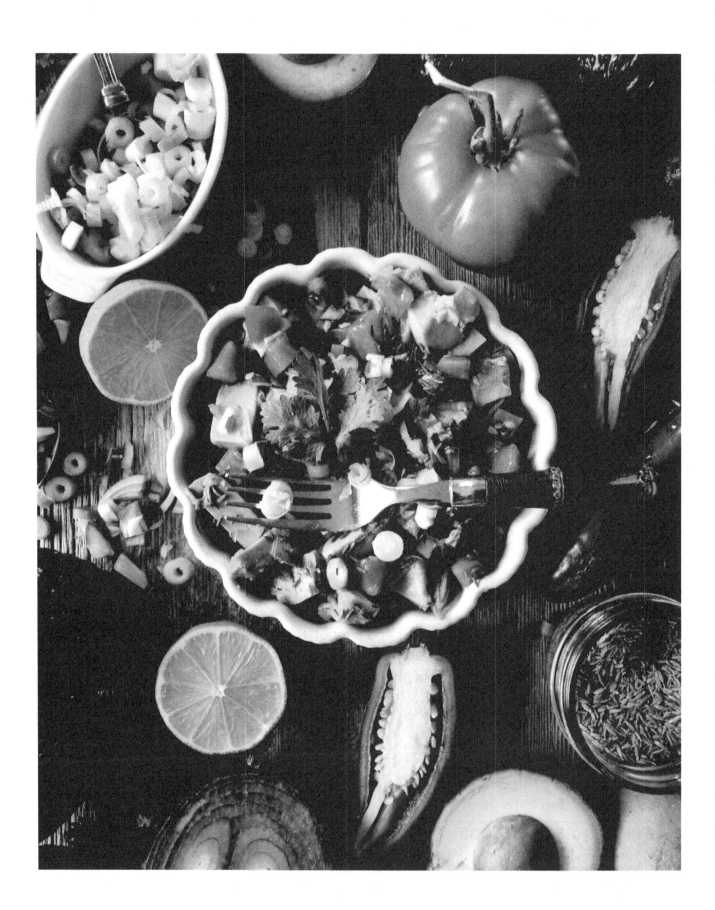

Chapter 8   VEGETABLES AND SALADS

1. Asian Pear Salad

2. Sesame Cucumber Salad

3. Fruity Zucchini Salad

4. Cranberry Frozen Salad

5. Waldorf Salad

6. Cucumber-Dill Cabbage Salad

7. Yellow Squash & Green Onions

8. Leaf Lettuce and Asparagus Salad with Raspberries

9. Fried Onion Rings

10. Bow-Tie Pasta Salad

11. Cottage Cheese Salad

12. Jicama and Carrot Slaw

13. Tortellini Salad

14. Fresh Sweet Corn Salad

15. Easy Avocado and Romaine Lettuce Salad

EAT YOUR GREENS, THEY ARE GOOD FOR YOU!

IN THIS CHAPTER, YOU WILL FIND A DIVERSE RANGE OF RECIPES THAT HIGHLIGHT THE NUTRITIONAL BENEFITS OF FRESH, KIDNEY-FRIENDLY VEGETABLES. FROM ASIAN PEAR SALAD TO FRESH SWEET CORN SALAD, THESE RECIPES ARE NOT ONLY TASTY BUT ALSO EASY TO PREPARE. GET INSPIRED TO INCORPORATE MORE VEGETABLES AND SALADS INTO YOUR RENAL DIET WITH THESE FLAVORFUL RECIPES.

1. ASIAN PEAR SALAD

Servings: 6   **Duration: 30 minutes**

INGREDIENTS	INSTRUCTIONS
<ul><li>¼ cup olive oil</li><li>2 cups green cabbage, shredded</li><li>1 Asian pear, cored and grated</li><li>1 cup red cabbage, shredded</li><li>Juice of 1 lime</li><li>2 celery stalks, chopped</li><li>½ red bell pepper, boiled and chopped</li><li>½ cup chopped cilantro</li><li>2 scallions, chopped</li><li>Zest of 1 lime</li><li>1 tsp granulated sugar</li></ul>	1. Mix the green and red cabbage, pear, scallions, red pepper, celery, and cilantro in a large bowl. 2. In another small bowl, whisk the olive oil, lime zest, lime juice, and sugar together. 3. Mix the dressing with the cabbage mixture. 4. Chill for an hour in the fridge before serving.

NUTRIENTS (PER SERVING):

Calories: 105 | Fat: 9g | Sodium: 48mg | Protein: 1g | Carbs: 6g | Phosphorus: 17mg | Potassium: 136mg

2. SESAME CUCUMBER SALAD

Servings: 4   **Duration: 25 minutes**

INGREDIENTS	INSTRUCTIONS
• 1 tbsp honey • 3-5 Persian cucumbers • 1 tbsp sesame seeds • 2 tbsp low sodium soy sauce • 1 bird's eye chili (optional) • 2 tbsp rice vinegar	1. Put the sesame seeds, soy sauce, rice vinegar and honey in a large bowl. Add the chopped chili (optional). If you want less spice, remove the seeds. 2. Thinly slice the cucumbers with a sharp knife. Thinner is better. 3. Assemble everything. 4. Let it set in the fridge for 20 minutes or longer.

NUTRIENTS (PER SERVING):

Calories: 140 | Carbs: 8g | Protein: 6g | Fiber: 2g | Fat: 2g | Vitamin C: 3mg |
Calcium: 37mg | Iron: 1mg | Sugar: 2g

3. FRUITY ZUCCHINI SALAD

Servings: 2   **Duration: 10 minutes**

INGREDIENTS	INSTRUCTIONS
• 200g (7oz) strawberries • 1 Tbsp honey • 1 cup cooked noodles • 1 big zucchini • 50g (1.7oz) dried cranberries/ raisins • 40g (1.4oz) almonds • 100g (3.5oz) blueberries • 1 tbsp lime juice	1. Assemble 1 tablespoon of honey with 1 tablespoon of lime juice in a bowl. 2. Mix the peeled and grated zucchini (or any desirable shapes) into the bowl of noodles with the lime dressing. 3. Add berries and almonds, stir and toss again to ensure everything is well mixed. Serve immediately!

NUTRIENTS (PER SERVING):

Calories: 202 | Carbs: 20g | Fiber: 6g | Protein: 7g | Fat: 9g

4. CRANBERRY FROZEN SALAD

Servings: 8   **Duration: 30 minutes**

INGREDIENTS	INSTRUCTIONS
• 1 16-oz can cranberry sauce • 1 8-oz package cream cheese • ½ pint whipping cream, whipped • ½ tsp vanilla extract	1. Use a mixer to make the cream cheese fluffy. Mix in vanilla, whipped cream, and cranberry sauce in that order. Assemble well. 2. Place mixture in a 9x9-inch greased pan. Freeze for 30 to 60 minutes or more. ***Serve frozen and cut into pretty slices. Enjoy healthy eating!***

NUTRIENTS (PER SERVING):
Calories: 255 | Carbs: 11g | Protein: 2.5g | Fat: 9g | Sodium: 99mg | Potassium: 63mg | Phosphorus: 46mg

5. WALDORF SALAD

Servings: 4   **Duration: 20 minutes**

INGREDIENTS	INSTRUCTIONS
• 3 celery stalks, chopped • 1 tbsp granulated sugar • 3 cups torn green leaf lettuce • 1 cup halved grapes • ½ cup light sour cream • 2 tbsp freshly squeezed lemon juice • 1 large apple, peeled and chopped	1. Put the lettuce on 4 plates in an even way, and set aside. 2. Mix the grapes, apple and celery together in a small bowl. 3. Mix sugar, lemon juice, and sour cream in another small bowl. 4. Mix the sour cream mixture and the grape mixture. 5. Place an equal amount of the grape mixture dressed with the sour cream mixture on each plate.

NUTRIENTS (PER SERVING):
Carbs: 15g | Potassium: 194mg | Phosphorus: 29mg | Sodium: 30mg | Protein: 1g | Fat: 2g

6. CUCUMBER-DILL CABBAGE SALAD

Servings: 4   **Duration: 25 minutes**

INGREDIENTS	INSTRUCTIONS
• 1 English cucumber, thinly sliced • 2 tbsp chopped fresh dill • ¼ cup heavy cream • 2 tbsp granulated sugar • ¼ tsp freshly ground black pepper • 2 cups shredded cabbage • 2 tbsp finely chopped scallion, green part only • ¼ cup freshly squeezed lemon juice	1. Mix the cream, lemon juice, sugar, dill, scallion, and pepper in a small bowl until well blended. 2. Combine the cucumber and cabbage in a large bowl. 3. Pour the lime dressing over the cucumber salad. 4. Put the salad in the fridge for an hour to chill. 5. Stir before serving.

NUTRIENTS (PER SERVING):
Calories: 99 | Fat: 6g | Protein: 2g | Carbs: 13g | Phosphorus: 38mg | Potassium: 200mg | Sodium: 14mg

7. YELLOW SQUASH & GREEN ONIONS

Servings: 4   **Duration: 15 minutes**

INGREDIENTS	INSTRUCTIONS
• 2 tbsp butter or margarine • 2 cups yellow straight neck washed and sliced • 1 cup green onion, chopped • Pinch of salt & black pepper	1. Boil the slices of squash for 15 minutes or until soft. Drain. 2. In a frying pan, melt butter add onion and Sauté until tender. 3. Add squash and black pepper to the pan and stir. 4. Now put a lid on it and let it cook on low heat for about 5 minutes. Serve hot sprinkle crumbed cheese if desired (optional). ***Serve with meat or over rice as a main vegetable.***

NUTRIENTS (PER SERVING):
Calories: 87 | Sodium: 347mg | Protein: 1.5g | Cholesterol: 0mg | Potassium: 204mg | Carbohydrate: 4g

8. LEAF LETTUCE AND ASPARAGUS SALAD WITH RASPBERRIES

Servings: 4   **Duration: 25 minutes**

INGREDIENTS	INSTRUCTIONS
• 1 cup raspberries • 1 cup asparagus, cut into long ribbons • 2 tbsp balsamic vinegar • Freshly ground black pepper • 1 scallion, both green and white parts, sliced • 2 cups shredded green leaf lettuce	1. Put equal amounts of lettuce on each of 4 plates. 2. Arrange the asparagus and scallions on top of the greens. 3. Place raspberries on top of the salads and spread evenly on each of the 4 plates. 4. Drizzle balsamic vinegar over the salads. 5. Add pepper to taste.

NUTRIENTS (PER SERVING):
Calories: 36 | Fat: 0g | Carbs: 8g | Phosphorus: 43mg | Sodium: 11mg | Protein: 2g

9. FRIED ONION RINGS

Servings: 4   **Duration: 30 minutes**

INGREDIENTS	INSTRUCTIONS
• 1 egg, beaten • ½ cup vegetable oil for frying • ¾ cup plain cornmeal • ¼ cup all-purpose flour • 4 medium onions • ¼ cup water • 1 tsp sugar	1. Mix together the flour, cornmeal, and sugar, and set it aside. 2. Peel the onions and cut them into slices about 14" thick. Isolate into rings. 3. Mix the beaten egg with the water. 4. Dip the rings in the egg wash and then in the cornmeal mix. 5. Fry rings in hot vegetable oil for 3 to 5 minutes, turning until brown. 6. Drain on a piece of paper towel. Serve warm.

NUTRIENTS (PER SERVING):
Carbs: 14 | Protein: 2g | Total Fat: 11g | Cholesterol: 27mg | Phosphorus: 39g | Fiber: 2g

10. BOW-TIE PASTA SALAD

Servings: 8   **Duration: 20 minutes**

INGREDIENTS	INSTRUCTIONS
• 1/4 cup chopped celery • 2 tbsp shredded carrot • 2/3 cup mayonnaise • 2 tbsp chopped green pepper • 1/2 tsp sugar • 1 tbsp lemon juice • 2 cups cooked bow-tie pasta • 2 tbsp minced onion • 1/8 tsp pepper	1. Mix 2 cups pasta, 2 tbsp green pepper, ¼ cup celery, 2 tbsp carrot, and 2 tbsp onion in a bowl. 2. Take another small bowl, and whisk together the pepper, mayonnaise, sugar, and lemon juice until smooth. 3. Pour mayonnaise mixture over the pasta and veggies and mix until everything is well coated. ***Serve chill or at room temperature.***

NUTRIENTS (PER SERVING):

Calories: 189 | Carbs: 12g | Fat: 15g | Sodium: 111mg | Phosphorus: 31mg | Protein: 2g | Potassium: 61mg

11. COTTAGE CHEESE SALAD

Servings: 11   **Duration: 20 minutes**

INGREDIENTS	INSTRUCTIONS
• 1 6-oz. can juice-packed crushed pineapple • 2 lb creamed cottage cheese • 1 3-oz package Jell-O® — raspberry • 1 8-oz carton whipped cream	1. Combine powdered Jell-O® with cottage cheese. Add the drained pineapple. 2. Mix the whipped cream in, toss and fold with a light hand until well combined. ***Sprinkle with salt and pepper if needed (optional). Chill and serve.***

NUTRIENTS (PER SERVING):

Calories: 191 | Carbs: 5g | Protein: 17g | Fat: 11g | Sodium: 348mg | Potassium: 105mg | Phosphorus: 122mg

12. JICAMA AND CARROT SLAW

Servings: 4-5   **Duration: 20 minutes**

INGREDIENTS	INSTRUCTIONS
• 1 pound jicama (about 2 large) • 3 tbsp cup olive oil • ½ cups pineapple juice • 1 tsp ground coriander • 1-pound carrots • ¼ cup fresh lime juice • Salt and pepper, to taste	1. Mix pineapple juice, lime juice, and oil in a bowl. Stir in pepper, salt, and coriander. 2. Now cut off the rough skin of the jicama and peel the carrots. Cut the jicama and carrots with a sharp knife in a matchstick shape about 3 inches long and 1/8 inch thick. 3. Mix the jicama and carrots in a large bowl, then pour the dressing on top. Assemble everything well and add more salt and pepper to taste (if needed). Serve!

NUTRIENTS (PER SERVING):

Calories: 53.9 | Carbs: 7g | Protein: 0.6g | Fat: 2g | Sodium: 52.2mg | Fiber: 2.8g

13. TORTELLINI SALAD

Servings: 4   **Duration: 30 minutes**

INGREDIENTS	INSTRUCTIONS
• 2 cups fresh arugula • 18 ounces cheese tortellini • 1 cup cooked white beans, drained and rinsed • 2 cups halved cherry tomatoes • 5 pepperoncini, stemmed and chopped • 1 cup fresh basil, torn • Italian Dressing • 1 14-ounce can artichoke hearts, drained and chopped • Red pepper flakes, optional • ½ cup thinly sliced red onion	1. Cook tortellini according to the directions on the package. When ready, drain the water and let it cool. 2. Mix the tortellini, tomatoes, artichokes, beans, onion, pepperoncini, and dressing together in a large bowl and toss to assemble. 3. Stir again after adding the arugula and basil. Pour Italian dressing and fold. Season to your taste; add Parmesan (optional) and red pepper flakes if you want. 4. ***Add more fresh basil to the top and serve right away.*** You can also store it in the fridge for up to 3 days.

NUTRIENTS (PER SERVING):

Protein: 6g | Carbs: 20g | Fat: 8g

14. FRESH SWEET CORN SALAD

Servings: 4   **Duration: 20 minutes**

INGREDIENTS	INSTRUCTIONS
• 2 tbsp basil for garnish, fresh thinly sliced • ¼ tsp ground pepper • 1 cup thinly sliced red onion • 1 tsp olive oil • 1 cup thin strips orange bell pepper • 4 medium ears fresh corn, boiled • ½ tsp kosher salt	1. Cut 2 cups of corn kernels off the cobs. 2. On medium heat, heat the oil in a 10-inch skillet. 3. Add the boiled soft corn, onion, and bell pepper. 4. Cook, stirring, for about 5 minutes or until the bell pepper and onion are soft but still crisp. Add salt and pepper to taste.

NUTRIENTS (PER SERVING):
Carbs: 21g | Fiber: 3g | Sodium: 155mg | Protein: 3g | Sugars: 8g

15. EASY AVOCADO AND ROMAINE LETTUCE SALAD

Servings: 4   **Duration: 20 minutes**

INGREDIENTS	INSTRUCTIONS
• 2 tbsp corn oil or avocado oil • ¼ tsp salt • 2 ripe avocados, diced • ¼ tsp ground pepper • 4 cups chopped romaine lettuce • 1 clove garlic, grated • 2 tbsp lime juice • 1 cup grape tomatoes, quartered	1. Mix the oil, lime juice, garlic, salt, and pepper in a large bowl. Let it sit for 3-4 minutes. 2. Now add the romaine, avocado, tomatoes, onion, and jalapeno, gently toss and fold.

NUTRIENTS (PER SERVING):
Calories: 245 | Carbs: 13.4g | Fiber: 8.4g | Potassium: 720.2mg | Sodium: 185.4mg | Protein: 3.1g

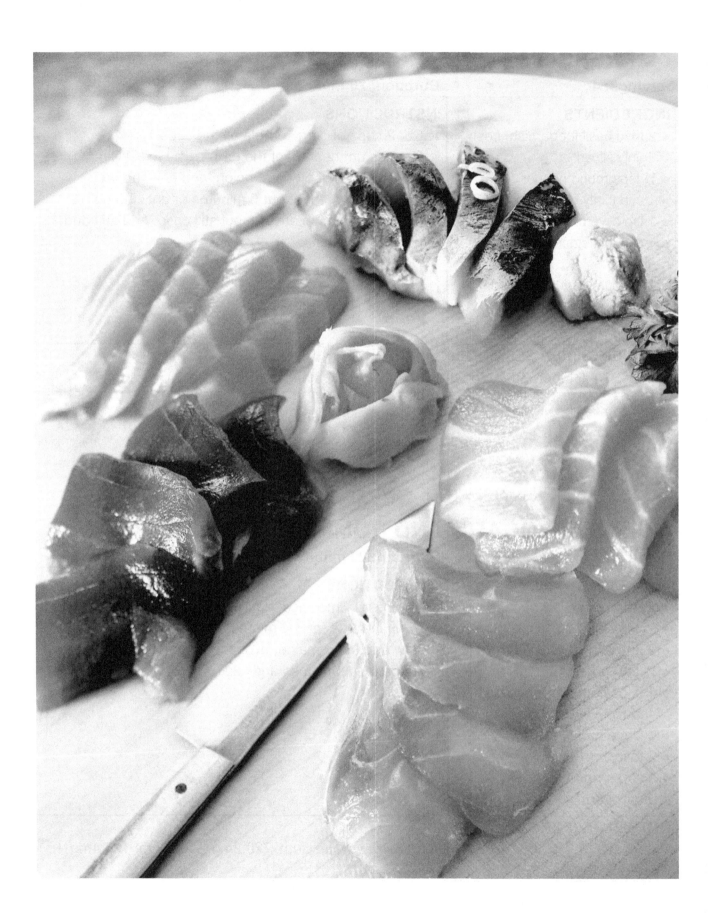

Chapter 9   FISH AND SEAFOOD

1. Salmon in Dill Sauce

2. Parmesan Baked Fish

3. Cod & Green Bean Risotto

4. Cod Peas

5. Shrimp Scampi Linguine

6. Broiled Garlic Shrimp

7. Baked Halibut

8. Scampi Linguini

9. Smoked Mackerel Paté

10. Crab Cakes

11. Fish Tacos

12. Sweet Glazed Salmon

13. Herb-Crusted Baked Haddock

14. Herb Pesto Tuna

15. Grilled Calamari with Lemon and Herbs

THERE ARE PLENTY OF FISH IN THE SEA!

IN THIS CHAPTER, YOU WILL FIND A VARIETY OF KIDNEY-FRIENDLY RECIPES THAT FEATURE THESE NUTRIENT-RICH FOODS. FROM SALMON IN DILL SAUCE TO GRILLED CALAMARI, THESE RECIPES ARE BOTH DELICIOUS AND EASY TO PREPARE. DISCOVER NEW WAYS TO INCORPORATE FISH AND SEAFOOD INTO YOUR RENAL DIET WITH THESE TASTY RECIPES.

1. SALMON IN DILL SAUCE

Servings: 6 **Duration: 35 minutes**

INGREDIENTS
- ¼ cup butter, cubed
- 1 tsp lemon-pepper seasoning
- 1 salmon fillet (about 2 pounds)
- 6 lemon slices
- 1 small onion, sliced
- 1 tsp onion salt

Dill Sauce:
- ⅓ cup mayonnaise
- ¼ tsp garlic salt
- ¾ tsp dill weed
- 1 tbsp finely chopped onion
- 1 tsp prepared horseradish
- ⅓ cup sour cream
- 1 tsp lemon juice
- Pepper to taste

INSTRUCTIONS
1. Line a 15x10x1-inch baking pan with heavy-duty foil and lightly grease. Place the salmon, skin side down, on the foil. Sprinkle with onion salt and lemon pepper.
2. Add onion and lemon to the top. Use butter to a dot. Fold foil around salmon and seal it tightly,
3. Bake for 20 minutes at 350°F. Carefully open the foil to let the steam out.
4. Broil the fish 4-6 inches from the heat for 3 to 5 minutes or until it flakes easily with a fork.
5. Mix the ingredients for the sauce together until smooth. Serve with salmon and enjoy!

NUTRIENTS (PER SERVING):
Carbs: 17g | Protein: 20g | Fiber: 1g | Fat: 0g | Cholesterol: 98mg

2. PARMESAN BAKED FISH

Servings: 8   **Duration: 35 minutes**

INGREDIENTS	INSTRUCTIONS
• ¼ tsp onion powder • 2 pounds fish fillets • 1/8 tsp paprika • ¼ tsp ground thyme • ¾ cup non-fat milk • ¾ cup plain bread crumbs • ¼ cup grated parmesan cheese	1. Turn the oven on to 500°F. 2. Spray some cooking spray on a baking sheet. 3. Mix the bread crumbs, Parmesan cheese, thyme, onion powder, and paprika in a small bowl. 4. Spread the crumb mixture out on a flat plate. Dip the fish fillets in milk, and then press all sides into the crumb mixture. 5. Place the fish in a single layer on the baking sheet. Depending on the fish's thickness, bake it for about 15 minutes or until it is opaque and flakes easily in the thickest part. Serve warm.

NUTRIENTS (PER SERVING):
Calories: 140 | Carbs: 7g | Protein: 14g | Fat: 2g | Sodium: 140mg | Cholesterol: 45mg

3. COD & GREEN BEAN RISOTTO

Servings: 4   **Duration: 20 minutes**

INGREDIENTS	INSTRUCTIONS
• 1 ¼ lb. skinless cod, cut into 4 pieces • ¼ cup grated Parmesan • 2 tbsp basil pesto • 1 lb. beans (green, wax or a combination) • Freshly ground black pepper • 2 tbsp extra-virgin olive oil • kosher salt	1. Heat oven to 425 degrees F. 2. On a large baking sheet with a rim, toss the beans with 1 tsp of oil, the Parmesan, and ¼ tsp each of salt and pepper. Roast for 8-10 minutes until golden brown. 3. In the meantime, put the remaining oil in a large skillet over medium flame. 4. Season each cod with ¼ tsp salt and pepper, then cook for about 3 minutes per side or until golden brown. Move the fish to plates. 5. Put the pesto on top of the cod and serve with the beans.

NUTRIENTS (PER SERVING):
Calories: 242 | Fat: 11g | Cholestrol: 61mg | Protein: 20g | Carbs: 10g | Fiber: 3g

4. COD PEAS

Servings: 4   **Duration: 12 minutes**

INGREDIENTS	INSTRUCTIONS
• 1 cup thawed frozen green peas • 4 (6-oz.) cod fillets • 2 tbsp lime juice • 2 tbsp capers • 2 tbsp olive oil • 2 tbsp chopped shallots • ¼ tsp crushed red pepper • 1 ½ tbsp chopped, fresh oregano • ½ tsp kosher salt • 1 tbsp olive oil	1. Mix together the peas, capers, oregano, shallots, lime juice, ¼ tsp of kosher salt, 2 tbsp of olive oil, and crushed red pepper. 2. Sprinkle ¼ tsp. kosher salt over cod fillets. 3. Heat a nonstick skillet over medium-high. Add 1 tbsp of olive oil and cod. Cook for 4 minutes per side or more until perfectly cooked. **Serve cod with peas on top.**

NUTRIENTS (PER SERVING):
Calories: 224 | Fat: 11g | Protein: 20g | Carbs: 7g | Fiber: 2g | Cholesterol: 67mg

5. SHRIMP SCAMPI LINGUINE

Servings: 4   **Duration: 15 minutes**

INGREDIENTS	INSTRUCTIONS
• 2 tsp minced garlic • 4 ounces uncooked linguine • 1 tsp olive oil • 1 lemon, juiced • Freshly ground black pepper • 4 ounces shrimp, peeled, deveined, and chopped • ½ cup (whipping) cream • 1 tbsp chopped fresh basil	1. Follow the package instructions to cook the linguine; drain it and set it aside. 2. Heat the olive oil in a large pan over medium heat. 3. Cook shrimp for about 6 minutes or until opaque. Sauté the garlic with the shrimp. 4. Add lemon juice and basil and cook for 5 minutes more. 5. Now mix in cream and cook for another 2 minutes. 6. When everything is well combined, put the linguine in the pan and toss to coat. 7. **Divide the pasta among 4 plates and serve.**

NUTRIENTS (PER SERVING):
Calories: 219 | Protein: 12g | Carbs: 21g | Fat: 7g | Phosphorus: 119mg | Potassium: 155mg | Sodium: 42mg

6. BROILED GARLIC SHRIMP

Servings: 4-5 **Duration: 25 minutes**

INGREDIENTS	INSTRUCTIONS
• 2 tbsp chopped onion • ½ cup unsalted margarine, melted • ⅛ tsp pepper • 1 tbsp fresh parsley, chopped • 1 clove garlic, minced • 2 tsp lemon juice • 1 lb. shrimp in shells	1. Heat the broiler. Clean, peel, and dry the shrimp. Put margarine in a shallow baking pan and add lemon juice, onion, garlic, and pepper. 2. Put in shrimp and stir to coat. 3. Broil for 5 minutes. 4. Flip and broil for 5 minutes more. Serve on a platter with the strained juices. Put some parsley on top.

NUTRIENTS (PER SERVING):
Calories: 264 | Carbs: 2g | Protein: 19g | Fat: 20g | Sodium: 135mg |
Phosphorus: 192mg

7. BAKED HALIBUT

Servings: 7 **Duration: 30 minutes**

INGREDIENTS	INSTRUCTIONS
• 1 ½ lb. halibut steaks • Lemon slices dipped in paprika • ¾ cup bread crumbs • ¼ cup mayonnaise	1. Turn oven on to 400°F. Cut steaks away from the bone in the middle and into serving-size pieces. Coat with mayonnaise. Roll in crumbs of bread. 2. Place in a greased baking dish. Bake in a preheated oven for approximately 15 minutes or until the fish flakes easily with a fork. 3. Place on a heated platter for serving. ***Add lemon slices to the top (optional). Enjoy!***

NUTRIENTS (PER SERVING):
Calories: 205 | Carbs: 8g | Protein: 22g | Fat: 9g | Sodium: 176mg | Potassium: 456mg

8. SCAMPI LINGUINI

Servings: 4   **Duration: 25 minutes**

INGREDIENTS	INSTRUCTIONS
• 1 clove garlic, minced • 1/2 lb. shrimp, peeled and cleaned • 1 tbsp olive oil • 1 tbsp chopped fresh parsley • 4 oz. dry linguini • 1/2 tsp basil • 1 tbsp lemon juice	1. Heat oil in a large skillet. Stir in shrimp and minced garlic. Stir shrimp while cooking until it turns pink. Add basil and parsley. 2. Cook for an extra 5 minutes. In the meantime, boil linguini in water without salt until it is soft. 3. Drain linguini. 4. Serve the linguini with the shrimp and the remaining liquid on top.

NUTRIENTS (PER SERVING):

Calories: 208 | Carbs: 19g | Protein: 15g | Fat: 5g | Sodium: 86mg | Potassium: 189mg

9. SMOKED MACKEREL PATÉ

Servings: 3-6   **Duration: 20 minutes**

INGREDIENTS	INSTRUCTIONS
• 200g (7oz) smoked mackerel fillets, skin removed • 1 tbsp creamed horseradish • 2 spring onions, trimmed and finely sliced • Pepper to taste • 100g (3½ oz) low-fat cream cheese • 1 lemon	1. Break the smoked mackerel into pieces and chop it up very small. Mix the mackerel, cream cheese, green onions, creamed horseradish, and the zest of one lemon together in a large bowl. 2. Squeeze the lemon juice into the mixture and mix until you have a thick paste. Season pepper and salt to taste. ***Enjoy this low-phosphate pate on toasted bread, Melba toast, or any other cracker.***

NUTRIENTS (PER SERVING):

Calories: 186 | Carbs: 2g | Protein: 21g | Fat: 10g | Sodium: 119mg |
Potassium: 232mg

10. CRAB CAKES

Servings: 6   **Duration: 30 minutes**

INGREDIENTS	INSTRUCTIONS
• 1 egg • 2 tbsp vegetable oil • ¼ cup reduced-fat mayonnaise • 1 tbsp dry mustard • ⅓ cup low-sodium crackers • 1 pound lump crab meat • ⅓ cup green or red pepper, finely chopped • 2 tbsp lemon juice • 1 tsp garlic powder • 1 tsp crushed red pepper or black pepper	1. Combine all the above ingredients in a large bowl except oil. 2. Assemble the ingredients well but do not shred the crab meat fully. Divide the material into 6 balls and shape patties. 3. Heat vegetable oil in a pan at low-medium flame. 4. Transfer the patties to the frying pan, fry and flip each side with 3 to 4 minutes gap. ***When done, serve warm with any green sauce.***

NUTRIENTS (PER SERVING):

Calories: 101 | Carbs: 5g | Phosphorus: 53mg | Fiber: 0g | Sodium: 67mg | Protein: 2g | Cholesterol: 42mg | Potassium: 72mg

11. FISH TACOS

Servings: 4   **Duration: 30 minutes**

INGREDIENTS	INSTRUCTIONS
• ¼ cup lemon juice • 1 tsp garlic powder • 12-16 fish fillets (1 pound), tilapia or as desired • ¼ cup unsalted butter • 20 saltine crackers, unsalted tops, crushed finely • 2 tsp dill weed	1. Turn the oven on to 400°F. 2. In a shallow pot, mix garlic and dill with crackers. Melt butter in another small bowl. 3. Roll the fish in melted butter, then in breadcrumbs, and then in the butter mixture again. 4. Place in a baking dish and bake for 8-10 minutes or until the fish flakes easily. ***Serve with avocado rice or any dish you desire.***

NUTRIENTS (PER SERVING):

Calories: 164 | Sodium: 138mg | Protein: 21g | Cholesterol: 57mg | Potassium: 335mg | Carbs: 7g | Phosphorus: 181mg | Fiber: 2g

12. SWEET GLAZED SALMON

Servings: 4   **Duration: 10 minutes**

INGREDIENTS	INSTRUCTIONS
• 4 (3-ounce) salmon fillets • ½ tsp freshly ground black pepper • ½ scallion, white and green parts, chopped • 1 tsp lemon zest • 2 tbsp honey • 1 tbsp olive oil • Salt to taste	1. Mix the honey, pepper, lemon zest, and salt in a small bowl. 2. Wash and dry the salmon with paper towels. 3. Cover each fillet with the honey mixture. You can keep the marinated salmon in the refrigerator for 1 hour (optional). 4. Heat the olive oil in a large pan over medium heat. 5. Add the salmon fillets and cook for approximately 10 minutes, flipping once or until the fish is lightly browned and cooked through. 6. Chop a scallion and sprinkle it on top. Serve!

NUTRIENTS (PER SERVING):

Calories: 240 | Carbs: 9g | Protein: 17g | Phosphorus: 205mg | Potassium: 317mg | Sodium: 51mg | Fat: 15g

13. HERB-CRUSTED BAKED HADDOCK

Servings: 4   **Duration: 10 minutes**

INGREDIENTS	INSTRUCTIONS
• ½ cup bread crumbs • ¼ tsp freshly ground black pepper • 12-ounce haddock fillets, deboned and skinned • 1 tsp chopped fresh thyme • 1 tbsp melted unsalted butter • 1 tbsp lemon zest • 3 tbsp chopped fresh parsley	1. Set the oven temperature to 350°F. 2. Mix the bread crumbs, parsley, lemon zest, thyme, and pepper together in a small bowl. 3. Now mix in melted butter after 5 minutes gap until the ingredients look like coarse crumbs. 4. Put the haddock on a baking sheet and spoon the breadcrumb mixture on top. Press down hard. 5. Bake the haddock in the oven for about 20 minutes, until the fish is just cooked and breaks into chunks when pressed.

NUTRIENTS (PER SERVING):

Calories: 143 | Fat: 4g | Protein: 16g | Carbs: 10g | Phosphorus: 216mg | Potassium: 285mg | Sodium: 281mg

14. HERB PESTO TUNA

Servings: 4   **Duration: 15 minutes**

INGREDIENTS	INSTRUCTIONS
• 1 tsp olive oil • 4 (3-ounce) yellow-fin tuna fillets • Freshly ground black pepper • One lemon, cut into 8 thin slices • ¼ cup Herb Pesto	1. Set the grill to medium-high heat. 2. Drizzle the olive oil over the fish and sprinkle pepper on each fillet. 3. Cook the fish on the grill for 4 minutes. 4. Turn the fish over and put herb pesto and lemon slices on top of each piece. 5. Now grill the tuna for 5 to 6 minutes more or until it is cooked to medium-well.

NUTRIENTS (PER SERVING):
Calories: 103 | Fat: 2g | Carbs: 0g | Phosphorus: 236mg | Potassium: 374mg | Sodium: 38mg | Protein: 21g

15. GRILLED CALAMARI WITH LEMON AND HERBS

Servings: 4   **Duration: 10 minutes**

INGREDIENTS	INSTRUCTIONS
• 2 tbsp olive oil • ½ pound cleaned calamari • 2 tbsp freshly squeezed lemon juice • Pinch freshly ground black pepper • 1 tbsp chopped fresh oregano • Pinch sea salt • 1 tbsp chopped fresh parsley • 2 tsp minced garlic • Lemon wedges, for garnish	1. Mix the olive oil, lemon juice, parsley, oregano, garlic, salt, and pepper together in a large bowl. 2. Stir the calamari in the bowl to coat it. 3. Cover the bowl and put it in the fridge for 1 hour to let the calamari marinate. 4. Set the grill to medium-high heat. 5. Grill the calamari turning once, until it is firm and clear for about 3 minutes. Serve with lemon wedges on top.

NUTRIENTS (PER SERVING):
Calories: 81 | Fat: 7g | Carbohydrates: 2g | Phosphorus: 128mg | Potassium: 160mg | Sodium: 67mg | Protein: 3g

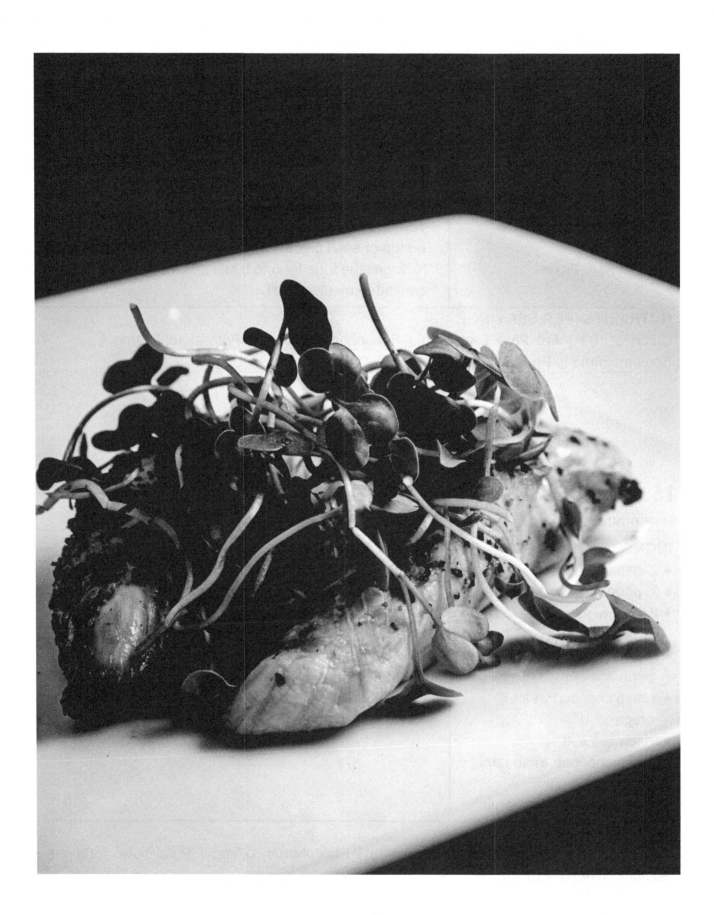

POULTRY

Chapter 10

1. Rosemary Chicken

2. Turkey & Sweet Potato Chili

3. Honey Garlic Chicken

4. Apricot Chicken Wings

5. Roasted Chicken Breast

6. Oven Fried Chicken

7. Indian Chicken Curry

8. Lemon Chicken

9. Chicken Stew

10. Persian Chicken

11. Chicken Fingers

12. Chicken Sausage Patties with Apple and Sage

13. Ground Chicken and Peas Curry

14. Herbed Chicken

15. Asian Chicken Satay

WINNER WINNER, CHICKEN DINNER!

IN THIS CHAPTER, YOU WILL FIND A VARIETY OF RECIPES THAT SHOWCASE THE VERSATILITY OF CHICKEN AND TURKEY IN A RENAL DIET. FROM ROSEMARY CHICKEN SKEWERS TO ASIAN CHICKEN SATAY, THESE RECIPES ARE BOTH FLAVORFUL AND KIDNEY FRIENDLY. LEARN HOW TO INCORPORATE POULTRY INTO YOUR RENAL DIET WITH THESE DELICIOUS AND EASY-TO-FOLLOW RECIPES.

1. ROSEMARY CHICKEN

Servings: 6   **Duration: 30 minutes**

INGREDIENTS	INSTRUCTIONS
• 3 large boneless, skinless chicken breasts • 3 tbsp butter • 3 tbsp fresh rosemary, chopped • ½ cup white vinegar • ¾ tsp pink peppercorns • 1 tsp salt • 3 cloves garlic • 1 cup dry vermouth • 1½ tbsp olive oil	1. Halve each chicken breast with a sharp knife. Use a paper towel to dry the chicken. 2. Heat a large skillet over medium-high heat. 3. Add the olive oil and butter. Once the butter has melted, add the whole garlic cloves and cook for 30 seconds to flavor the butter. Discard the garlic once it turns golden. 4. Add the chicken breasts and cook on each side for 1-2 minutes until nicely browned. 5. Lower heat to medium and add vinegar and salt. Cover and Simmer for 5 minutes until the vinegar has reduced, and the smell has dissipated. 6. Add in chopped rosemary and vermouth. Cook chicken uncovered until tender and 165 degrees Fahrenheit on a thermometer (about 10 minutes). Transfer chicken to a large serving platter. 7. Put the peppercorns in the skillet and bring the sauce to a boil. Boil for 3–5 minutes to reduce and thicken the sauce. Pour over the chicken and serve.

NUTRIENTS (PER SERVING):
Calories: 187 | Cholesterol: 56mg | Sodium: 183mg | Carbs: 0.9g | Fiber: 0.2g | Protein: 13g

2. TURKEY & SWEET POTATO CHILI

Servings: 8   **Duration: 50 minutes**

INGREDIENTS	INSTRUCTIONS
• 1 tbsp oil • 4 cups peeled, diced sweet potato (approximately 2 lbs.) • 3 tbsp chili powder • 2 tsp ground cumin • 3 (15 oz) cans fire-roasted diced tomatoes • 1 tsp ground coriander (or dried cilantro) • 1 tbsp onion powder • 1 (16 oz) package ground turkey • 2 tsp garlic powder • 2 tsp salt • 1 (28 oz) can crushed tomatoes • 1 tsp black pepper	1. In a large pot, heat oil over medium-high heat. 2. Add the ground turkey and cook until it turns brown, breaking up any big chunks. 3. Add the chili powder, cumin, coriander, onion powder, garlic powder, salt, and pepper. Saute for 1 minute, stirring constantly. 4. Stir in diced tomatoes, crushed tomatoes, and diced sweet potatoes. 5. Reduce the heat to low and let the sweet potatoes simmer for 30 minutes or until softened. ***Serve with optional toppings, such as diced avocado, sour cream, or shredded cheese.***

NUTRIENTS (PER SERVING):
Calories: 306 | Cholesterol: 60mg | Sodium: 209mg | Carbs: 31g | Fiber: 7g | Sugar: 8g | Protein: 13g

3. HONEY GARLIC CHICKEN

Servings: 6   **Duration: 45 minutes**

INGREDIENTS	INSTRUCTIONS
• ½ cup honey • 2-3 tsp canola oil, for frying • 6 chicken legs • 1 ¼" thick slice red onion, finely chopped • 2 slices ginger, cut to matchstick size • 2 garlic cloves, minced	1. Fry each side of the chicken legs for 7 minutes in a pan. 2. Take out and put in a casserole dish. Put the chopped onion, ginger matchsticks, minced garlic, and 1 tsp of oil in another frying pan. For 1 minute, fry. 3. Deglaze the pan by adding honey to the mixture and stirring it. Pour the sauce over the chicken and cook at 350° F for 35 minutes. ***Serve the prepared chicken on your favorite platter and enjoy!***

NUTRIENTS (PER SERVING):
Calories: 221 | Fat: 21g | Carbs: 5g | Phosphorus: 112mg | Potassium: 210mg | Sodium: 86mg | Protein: 2g

4. APRICOT CHICKEN WINGS

Servings: 4   **Duration: 45 minutes**

INGREDIENTS	INSTRUCTIONS
• 1 garlic clove, minced • 2 tbsp cider vinegar • 1 tsp chili powder • 1 cup apricot preserves • 2 pounds chicken wings with bones • 2 tsp hot pepper sauce (you can use any brand)	1. Cut each wing into three pieces and throw away the tips. Mix the remaining ingredients together in a small bowl, then pour 1/2 cup into a large resealable plastic bag. 2. Add the chicken, close the bag, and turn it to coat. 3. Refrigerate for at least 4 hours or overnight, turning the bag occasionally. Cover and put the rest of the marinade in the fridge. 4. Discard the marinade. Put the wings in a greased 15x10x1-inch pan lined with foil. 5. Bake at 400° for 30–35 minutes, or until the juices run clear, occasionally turning the chicken, and basting it with the remaining marinade.

NUTRIENTS (PER SERVING):

Calories: 57 | Cholesterol: 18mg | Sodium: 58mg | Carbs: 7g | Protein: 4g

5. ROASTED CHICKEN BREAST

Servings: 12   **Duration: 1 hour**

INGREDIENTS	INSTRUCTIONS
• 1 tbsp. McCormick No Salt Added Table shake seasoning® • 2 tbsp. olive oil • 2 tbsp. white vinegar • 4 chicken breasts (about 1 lb/500g) • 24 bamboo skewers	1. Cut the chicken into 24 thin strips 1 cm (1/2 inch) wide. 2. Mix oil, vinegar, and McCormick No Salt Added Table Shake Seasoning in a medium bowl. 3. Add strips of chicken and stir to coat. Cover and put in the fridge for at least 30 minutes or overnight, turning the meat occasionally. 4. For the next 30 minutes, soak bamboo skewers in water. 5. Take the chicken from the marinade and put one piece on each skewer. Grill or broil for about 5 min per side or until no longer pink. Discard any leftover marinade.

NUTRIENTS (PER SERVING):

Calories: 186 | Carbs: 2g | Fat: 10g | Sodium: 119mg | Potassium: 232mg | Protein: 1g

6. OVEN FRIED CHICKEN

Servings: 10   **Duration: 1 hour**

INGREDIENTS	INSTRUCTIONS
• ½ tsp onion powder • ¼ cup shortening • 1 3-lb broiled-fryer chicken, cut up • 1 tsp paprika • ½ cup flour • ¼ cup margarine • ½ tsp pepper	1. Preheat the oven to 425°F. Wash and dry the chicken. 2. Melt the shortening and margarine in a 13 x 9 x 2 inches baking pan in the oven. Mix the flour, paprika, pepper, and onion powder in a medium bowl. 3. Coat each piece of chicken with the flour mixture. 4. Put the skin side down of the chicken in the melted shortening for 30 minutes with the lid off. 5. Turn the chicken over and cook for another 30 minutes until the thickest pieces are fork tender.

NUTRIENTS (PER SERVING):
Calories: 186 | Carbs: 2g | Protein: 21g | Fat: 10g | Sodium: 119mg |
Potassium: 232mg

7. INDIAN CHICKEN CURRY

Servings: 6   **Duration: 20 minutes**

INGREDIENTS	INSTRUCTIONS
• 3 tbsp olive oil, divided • 6 boneless, skinless chicken thighs • 1 small sweet onion • 2 tsp minced garlic • 1 tsp grated fresh ginger • 1 tbsp Hot Curry Powder (here) • ¾ cup water • ¼ cup coconut milk • 2 tbsp chopped fresh cilantro	1. Heat 2 tbsp of the oil in a large pan over medium-high heat. 2. Add the chicken and cook for about 10 minutes until all sides of the thighs are browned. Put the chicken on a plate with tongs and set it aside. 3. Add the last tbsp of oil to the pan and cook the onion, garlic, and ginger for about 3 minutes or until soft. 4. Mix well with the curry powder, water, and coconut milk. 5. Bring the liquid to a boil, then return the chicken to the pan. 6. Reduce heat, cover the skillet, and let it simmer for about 25 minutes, or until the chicken is soft and the sauce is thick. ***Serve in your favorite dish with cilantro on top.***

NUTRIENTS (PER SERVING):
Calories: 241 | Fat: 14g | Carbs: 2g | Phosphorus: 145mg | Potassium: 230mg |
Sodium: 76mg | Protein: 26g

8. LEMON CHICKEN

Servings: 8   **Duration: 35 minutes**

INGREDIENTS	INSTRUCTIONS
• 1 tbsp lemon juice • 2 ½ pound fryer (cut as desired) • 1 cup cornflakes, crushed • 4 tbsp vegetable oil • 1 tsp black pepper • 1 cup all-purpose flour • ¼ tsp poultry seasoning	1. Preheat the oven to 400ºFWash the chicken parts well and pat dry; rub with lemon juice. 2. Put flour, black pepper, cornflakes, and poultry seasoning in a small bag and shake it well. Mix well. 3. Use vegetable oil to grease a shallow baking pan (about 1" deep). 4. Put the chicken in the bag with the other ingredients, starting with the biggest pieces. Mix well. 5. Put coated chicken in the pan. Brown in the oven for 20-30 minutes on each side.

NUTRIENTS (PER SERVING):
Calories: 280 | Sodium: 74mg | Protein: 15g | Cholesterol: 52g | Potassium: 150g | Carbs: 15g | Phosphorus: 120mg | Fiber: 1g

9. CHICKEN STEW

Servings: 6   **Duration: 45 minutes**

INGREDIENTS	INSTRUCTIONS
• 2 pounds chicken breast cut into bite-size pieces • 1 110-ounce bag frozen sliced okra • 1 cup sliced onions • 2 10 ½-ounce cans low-sodium chicken broth • 2 cloves garlic, minced • 1 10-ounce bag frozen carrots • 3 tbsp vegetable oil • ¾ cup green peppers • ¼ tsp dried basil • ¼ tsp black pepper • 2 tbsp all-purpose flour	1. In a dutch oven, heat 2 tablespoons of oil. Add the chicken and cook it over medium-high heat. 2. Remove the chicken and set it aside. Add the last tsp of oil. Put in onion, pepper, and garlic. 3. Add the flour and stir constantly for two to three minutes. Cook the chicken and broth until the water boils. 4. Add carrots, basil, and black pepper, cover, and let simmer for about 10 minutes. 5. As gravy cooks, it will get thicker. Add the okra and continue cooking for 5–10 minutes. ***Serve hot white rice on the side.***

NUTRIENTS (PER SERVING):
Calories: 142 | Sodium: 93mg | Protein: 10g | Cholesterol: 15mg | Carbs: 13g | Phosphorus: 123mg | Fiber: 3g

10. PERSIAN CHICKEN

Servings: 5   **Duration: 20 minutes (1 hour for marinating)**

INGREDIENTS	INSTRUCTIONS
• 1 tsp minced garlic • ½ small sweet onion, chopped • 1 tbsp dried oregano • ½ cup olive oil • 1 tsp sweet paprika • ½ tsp ground cumin • 5 boneless, skinless chicken thighs • ¼ cup freshly squeezed lemon juice	1. Mix the onion, lemon juice, oregano, garlic, paprika, and cumin using a blender. 2. Mix the ingredients by pulsing a few times. 3. Add the olive oil while the motor is running until the mixture is smooth. 4. Put the chicken thighs in a large, sealable freezer bag and pour the marinade into the bag. 5. Seal the bag and put it in the refrigerator, turning it twice for 2 hours. 6. Take the thighs out of the bag and leave the rest marinade. 7. Set the grill to medium heat. 8. The chicken must be on the grill for about 20 minutes, with one turn, or until the temperature inside is 165°F.

NUTRIENTS (PER SERVING):
Calories: 321 | Fat: 21g | Carbs: 3g | Phosphorus: 131mg | Potassium: 220mg | Sodium: 86mg | Protein: 22g

11. CHICKEN FINGERS

Servings: 12 chicken fingers   **Duration: 30 minutes**

INGREDIENTS	INSTRUCTIONS
• 4 chicken breasts (halves), boneless, skinless (cut into 1" strips) • ¾ cup breadcrumbs • ¼ tsp pepper • ¾ tsp each garlic & onion powder • 2 tbsp parmesan cheese • ¼ cup non-hydrogenated margarine, melted • 1 ½ tsp dried thyme	1. 1. Preheat oven to 400°F. Combine breadcrumbs, parmesan, 1 tsp pepper, 1 ½ tsp thyme, ¾ tsp garlic and onion powder. 2. Dip chicken into melted margarine; then coat with mixed ingredients. Place on a lightly greased rack on a cookie sheet. 3. Bake for 10 minutes, turn and bake 10 minutes more. ***Couple with your favorite sauce and serve warm!***

NUTRIENTS (PER FINGER):
Calories: 143 | Fat: 13g | Carbs: 7g | Phosphorus: 172mg | Potassium: 230mg | Sodium: 92mg | Protein: 1g

12. CHICKEN SAUSAGE PATTIES WITH APPLE AND SAGE

Servings: 4   **Duration: 30 minutes**

INGREDIENTS	INSTRUCTIONS
• 1 apple • 2 tbsp fresh sage or 2 tsp. dried • 1 egg, lightly beaten • ¼ tsp ground allspice • 2 cloves garlic, minced • 1 lb ground chicken • 1 cup minced onion • 1 tsp pepper	1. Grate the apple with the skin on and stir with onion, sage, allspice, garlic, pepper, and a beaten egg. 2. Stir the ground chicken until it is well-mixed. Make a log, wrap it in wax paper, and put it in the fridge for at least two hours or overnight. 3. Chilling the patties helps to keep their shape while cooking. 4. Cut the log into eight pieces and flatten each piece into a patty that is ½" thick. 5. Pan-fry the patties in a non-stick pan over medium heat for 6 minutes per side.

NUTRIENTS (PER SERVING) 2 PATTIES:
Calories: 132 | Fat: 19g | Carbs: 6g | Phosphorus: 143mg | Potassium: 230mg | Sodium: 86mg | Protein: 7g

13. GROUND CHICKEN AND PEAS CURRY

Servings: 4   **Duration: 20 minutes**

INGREDIENTS	INSTRUCTIONS
• 1 pound Ground Chicken • 1/3 cup (80g) Sweet Chili Sauce • 2 tbsp (30g) Chili Garlic Sauce • 1 packet Thai Curry peas* • 1 tbsp (15g) Low Sodium Soy Sauce • 1/2 tbsp (8g) Olive Oil • 1/2 tsp Ground Ginger • 1/2 tsp Kosher Salt • 15 oz. can Lite Coconut Milk	1. Heat a large skillet over medium-high heat. When the oil is hot, add the ground chicken. 2. Cook for 4 to 5 minutes until the bottom side is golden brown, then flip and brown the other side. 3. Use a spatula to pull the chicken apart and cook it through. 4. Once the meat is done, add everything else except the peas. 5. Add the peas, stir well, and bring to a boil, then reduce the heat, and cover for 10–12 minutes, or until very little liquid is left. (It should not be dry; it should still be a little creamy.) 6. Garnish with cilantro, roasted peanuts, lime wedges, and chili oil (such as chili garlic crisp), if desired.

NUTRIENTS (PER SERVING):
Calories: 415 | Total Fat: 14g | Carbs: 27g | Fiber: 9g | Protein: 16g

14. HERBED CHICKEN

Servings: 4   **Duration: 35 minutes**

INGREDIENTS	INSTRUCTIONS
• 2 tbsp. herbed seasoned flour • ½ cup low-sodium chicken stock • 4 chicken breasts (fresh) • 2 tbsp. butter **Herbed-Spiced Flour:** • 2 tsp. basil • 1 tsp paprika • 1 tsp tarragon • 2 tsp thyme • 1 tsp oregano • ½ cup flour • ½ tsp black pepper	1. 1. Coat the chicken with spiced flour. 2. Melt the butter in a large frying pan and brown the chicken on each side for 3 to 5 minutes. 3. Pour in the chicken stock and cook, stirring until it gets thicker. 4. Reduce the heat to medium and cover the chicken. Cook for 3–4 minutes on each side until the chicken is no longer pink.

NUTRIENTS (PER SERVING):
Calories: 123 | Protein: 3g | Carbs: 11g | Fat: 9g | Phosphorus: 112mg |
Potassium: 134mg | Sodium: 92mg

15. ASIAN CHICKEN SATAY

Servings: 6   **Duration: 15 minutes (1 hour for marinating)**

INGREDIENTS	INSTRUCTIONS
• 12 ounces boneless, skinless chicken breast, cut into 12 strips • Juice of 2 limes • 1 tbsp minced garlic • 2 tsp ground cumin • 2 tbsp brown sugar	1. Mix the lime juice, brown sugar, garlic, and cumin in a large bowl. 2. Put the chicken strips in the bowl and marinate for an hour in the fridge. 3. Set the grill to medium-high heat. 4. Take the chicken out of the marinade and put each strip on a skewer made of wood soaked in water. 5. Cook the chicken on the grill for about 4 minutes per side or until the meat is done but still juicy. ***Serve with rice pilaf or any green salad. Enjoy!***

NUTRIENTS (PER SERVING):
Calories: 78 | Fat: 2g | Carbs: 4g | Protein: 12g | Phosphorus: 116mg |
Potassium: 208mg | Sodium: 100mg

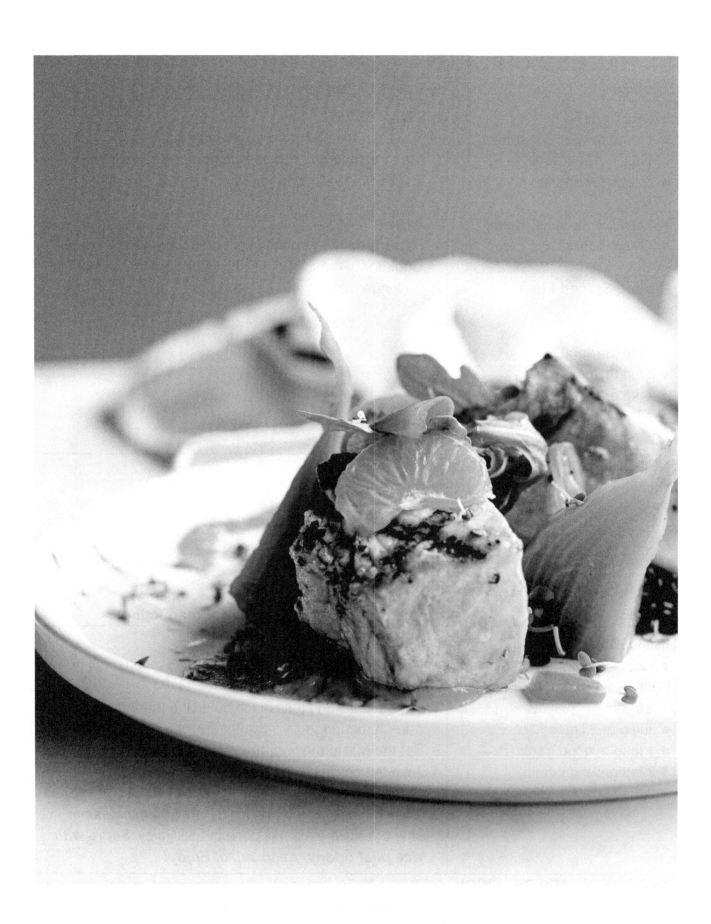

MEAT RECIPES

Chapter 11

1. Pork with Bell Pepper

2. Spicy Lamb Curry

3. Grilled Lamb Chops

4. Chinese Beef Wraps

5. Roast Beef

6. Open-Faced Beef Stir-Up

7. Sweet and Sour Meat Loaf

8. Grilled Steak

9. Onion Smothered Steak

10. Salisbury Steak

11. Swedish Meatballs

12. Taco Stuffing

13. Classic Pot Roast

14. Grilled Marinated Beef Steaks

15. Pan-Fried Pork Chop with Creamy Leek Sauce

MEAT IS NOT JUST FOOD, IT IS AN EMOTION THAT BRINGS PEOPLE TOGETHER.

IN THIS CHAPTER, YOU WILL FIND A RANGE OF RECIPES THAT INCORPORATE MEAT INTO A KIDNEY-FRIENDLY DIET. FROM CHINESE BEEF WRAPS TO GRILLED MARINATED BEEF STEAKS, THESE RECIPES ARE BOTH HEARTY AND NUTRITIOUS. DISCOVER NEW WAYS TO INCORPORATE MEAT INTO YOUR RENAL DIET WITH THESE DELICIOUS AND EASY-TO-FOLLOW RECIPES.

1. PORK WITH BELL PEPPER

Servings: 4   **Duration: 40 minutes**

INGREDIENTS	INSTRUCTIONS
• 6 cloves garlic, smashed • 1 large pork tenderloin (about 11/2 pounds), trimmed • 1 small onion, thickly sliced • 3 tbsp extra-virgin olive oil • 16 fresh sage leaves • 2 red and yellow bell peppers sliced into wide strips • ¼ cup sliced pickled pepperoncini, plus 2 tsp liquid from the jar • ⅔ cup low-sodium chicken broth • Kosher salt • 2 tbsp tomato paste • ¼ cup grated Parmesan	1. Get the broiler ready. Cut the pork into 1-inch thick and 1-inch-wide pieces and salt them. Put 1 tbsp of olive oil in a large oven-safe pan and heat it over medium-high heat. 2. Add the onion and bell peppers, sprinkle with ½ tsp of salt, and cook for 4 to 6 minutes, until the vegetables are crisp-tender and slightly browned. Put it onto a plate. 3. Put the last 2 tbsp of oil into the pan. Add the pork and sear it over high heat for 2 to 4 minutes per side until it is browned. Add the onion and peppers to the plate with the pork. 4. Turn the heat low to medium and stir in the garlic, sage, and tomato paste. Cook and stir the tomato paste for about a minute until it turns brick red. Add the pepperoncini slices and liquid. Bring to a boil and use a wooden spoon or spatula to scrape up any browned bits. 5. Add the broth and reduce the flame to low. Spread the pork out in a single layer in the pan. Add onion and peppers, and then sprinkle the cheese on top. Move the pork to the oven and broil for 4 to 7 minutes or until it is fully cooked. ***Serve hot on a platter with salad dressing.***

NUTRIENTS (PER SERVING):

Calories: 298 | Fat: 3g | Carbs: 13g | Phosphorus: 211mg | Potassium: 231mg | Sodium: 134mg | Protein: 11g

2. SPICY LAMB CURRY

Servings: 6 **Duration: 1 hour 30 minutes**

INGREDIENTS	INSTRUCTIONS
• 2 large garlic cloves, crushed • 6 lamb chops, about 3/4-inch thick • 1 tbsp fresh rosemary leaves • Pinch cayenne pepper • 2 tbsp extra-virgin olive oil • 1 tsp fresh thyme leaves • Coarse sea salt	1. Put the garlic, rosemary, thyme, cayenne, and salt in a food processor with a metal blade. Pulse until combined. 2. Pour olive oil in and pulse until it becomes a paste. Spread the paste on both sides of the lamb chops and put them in the fridge for at least an hour. 3. Take the chops from the fridge and let warm up to room temperature. This will take about 20 minutes. 4. When the chops are almost smoking, add them to a grill pan on high heat and grill for about 2 minutes. Turn the chops over and cook for 3 minutes for medium-rare or 3 1/2 minutes for medium. ***Serve the lamb curry with salad or any dressing and enjoy!***

NUTRIENTS (PER SERVING):
Calories: 203 | Protein: 30.7g | Carbs: 0.1g | Fiber: 0.1g | Fat: 7.9g | Cholesterol: 96.1mg | Potassium: 347mg | Sodium: 85mg

3. GRILLED LAMB CHOPS

Servings: 4 (3-ounce per-serving size) **Duration: 1 hour 30 minutes**

INGREDIENTS	INSTRUCTIONS
• 3 tsp dry mustard • 1 leg of lamb (trimmed for roasting) • ¼ cup vegetable oil • 1 ½ tbsp garlic powder	1. Mix the oil, garlic powder, and mustard for the marinade. 2. Marinate the lamb leg for 6–8 hours or overnight in the fridge. 3. Adjust the meat on the barbecue spit by positioning rightly over the roasted pan and roast for 30 minutes per pound. 4. Stirring the meat with the marinade constantly. When done, ***serve with lime juice and cilantro leaves on top***.

NUTRIENTS (PER SERVING):
Calories: 298 | Sodium: 144mg | Protein: 24g | Cholesterol: 73mg | Potassium: 423mg | Carbs: 3g | Phosphorus: 237mg

4. CHINESE BEEF WRAPS

Servings: 4   **Duration: 45 minutes**

INGREDIENTS	INSTRUCTIONS
• 4 garlic cloves • 1 tsp dark sesame oil • 1 medium cucumber • 1 pound ground beef • 1 cup rice, cooked • 1 tsp ground ginger • 8 pieces iceberg lettuce leaves, whole • 1 tbsp reduced-sodium soy sauce • 2 tsp red chili sauce • 1 medium red bell pepper • 2 tsp packed brown sugar	1. Chop garlic. Chop cucumber and bell pepper. 2. In a medium bowl, mix in ground meat with the garlic, soy sauce, red chili sauce, brown sugar, and ginger until well mixed. 3. Spray a large skillet with nonstick spray and put it over medium heat. 4. Add the beef mixture and cook it, breaking it up with a wooden spoon, until it has done (about three minutes). 5. Add the sesame oil and keep the beef warm. Warm up the rice. 6. In a bowl, mix the cucumber and the red bell pepper. 7. Fill each lettuce leaf with 1/4 cup of ground beef, 1/4 cup of the cucumber/red pepper mixture, and 2 tbsp cooked rice. ***Wrap and enjoy!***

NUTRIENTS (PER SERVING):

Calories: 308 | Protein: 26g | Carbs: 17g | Fat: 15g | Cholesterol: 77mg |
Sodium: 211mg | Potassium: 391mg | Fiber: 1.1g

5. ROAST BEEF

Servings: 6   **Duration: 1 hour (3 hours for marinating)**

INGREDIENTS	INSTRUCTIONS
• 2 tsp chili powder • 2 tbsp olive oil • 1-pound boneless pork leg roast • Pinch cayenne pepper • 2 tsp ground allspice • 1 tsp garlic powder • 1 tsp ground cinnamon • 1½ tsp ground cumin • ½ tsp freshly ground black pepper	1. Mix the chili powder, allspice, cumin, cinnamon, garlic powder, black pepper, and cayenne pepper together in a small bowl. 2. Rub the spice mixture all over the pork leg. Put the pork loin in the fridge for 3 hours to marinate. 3. Set the oven temperature to 350°F. Heat the olive oil in a large pan over medium-high heat. Cook the pork loin on all sides, then place it in an oven-safe dish. 4. Roast, uncovered, for about 40 minutes, or until the temperature inside reaches 160°F. Take the pork out of the oven and let it sit for 10 minutes. 5. To serve, cut the meat into thin slices.

NUTRIENTS (PER SERVING):

Calories: 98 | Fat: 4g | Carbs: 1g | Phosphorus: 130mg | Potassium: 240mg |
Sodium: 29mg | Protein: 13g

6. OPEN-FACED BEEF STIR-UP

Servings: 6 **Duration: 20 minutes**

INGREDIENTS	INSTRUCTIONS
• ½ cup shredded cabbage • ½ cup chopped sweet onion • 6 hamburger buns, bottom halves only • ½ pound 95% lean ground beef • ¼ cup Herb Pesto	1. In a large skillet, cook the beef and onion over medium heat for about 6 minutes or until the meat is done. 2. Add the cabbage and continue cooking for 3 more minutes. Add the pesto and cook for one minute. 3. Divide the beef mixture into 6 pieces and serve each on the open-faced hamburger buns bottom half. ***Enjoy and serve with your favorite drinks.***

NUTRIENTS (PER SERVING):

Calories: 120 | Fat: 3g | Carbs: 13g | Phosphorus: 106mg | Potassium: 198mg | Sodium: 134mg | Protein: 11g

7. SWEET AND SOUR MEAT LOAF

Servings: 8 **Duration: 1 hour**

INGREDIENTS	INSTRUCTIONS
• 1 large egg • 1 pound 95% lean ground beef • ½ cup bread crumbs • 1 tbsp brown sugar • ½ cup chopped sweet onion • 1 tsp white vinegar • 1 tsp chopped fresh thyme • ¼ tsp freshly ground black pepper • 2 tbsp chopped fresh basil • ¼ tsp garlic powder • 1 tsp chopped fresh parsley	1. Set the oven temperature to 350°F. 2. Mix the beef, bread crumbs, onion, egg, basil, thyme, parsley, and pepper until everything is well-mixed. 3. Press the meat mixture into a loaf pan that is 9 inches by 5 inches. 4. Mix brown sugar, vinegar, and garlic powder together in a small bowl. 5. Spread the brown sugar mixture over the meat in an even layer. 6. Bake the meatloaf for about 50 minutes or until it is cooked through. Let the meatloaf sit for 10 minutes, then pour out any grease that has built up. Serve hot!

NUTRIENTS (PER SERVING):

Calories: 103 | Fat: 3g | Carbs: 7g | Phosphorus: 112mg | Potassium: 190mg | Sodium: 87mg | Protein: 11g

8. GRILLED STEAK

Servings: 4   **Duration: 35 minutes**

INGREDIENTS
- 3 tbsp olive oil
- 4 (3-ounce) beef tenderloin steaks
- Freshly ground black pepper

INSTRUCTIONS
1. Set a grill to medium-high heat.
2. Take the steaks out of the fridge and let them sit at room temperature for about 10 minutes.
3. Spread olive oil all over the steaks and sprinkle with pepper.
4. Grill the steaks for about 5 minutes per side for medium-rare or until doneness you like.
5. *Serve the salsa on top of the steaks (optional).*

NUTRIENTS (PER SERVING):
Calories: 130 | Fat: 6g | Carbs: 1g | Phosphorus: 186mg | Potassium: 272mg | Sodium: 39mg | Protein: 19g

9. ONION SMOTHERED STEAK

Servings: 8 (2 oz. per serving)   Duration: 1 hour 20 minutes

INGREDIENTS
- ⅛ tsp pepper
- 1 clove garlic, minced
- 2 tbsp oil
- ¼ tsp dried thyme, crushed
- 1 tbsp vinegar
- ¼ cup flour
- 1 ½ lb round steak, 3/4-inch thick
- 1 bay leaf
- 1 cup water
- 3 medium onions, sliced

INSTRUCTIONS
1. Cut the steak into 8 equal pieces. Assemble the pepper and flour together, and then pound the meat.
2. In a pan, heat the oil and brown the meat on both sides. Remove from skillet and set aside.
3. Mix water, vinegar, bay leaf, garlic, and thyme in the pan. Bring it to a boil.
4. Put the meat in this mixture, and then top with sliced onions. Cover and let cook for an hour.

NUTRIENTS (PER SERVING):
Calories: 271 | Carbs: 7g | Protein: 18g | Fat: 19g | Sodium: 45mg | Potassium: 369mg

10. SALISBURY STEAK

Servings: 4   **Duration: 30 minutes**

INGREDIENTS	INSTRUCTIONS
• ½ cup water • 1 pound chopped steak • 1 egg • 1 tbsp vegetable oil • ½ cup green pepper, chopped • 1 small onion, chopped • 1 tbsp cornstarch • 1 tsp black pepper	1. Combine the meat, onion, black pepper, green pepper and egg in a shallow bowl. Form into patties. 2. Heat the oil in a large skillet, add the patties, and cook on both sides. 3. Add half the water and cook for 15 minutes on low heat. Exclude patties. 4. Add the rest of the water and cornstarch to the meat drippings. Simmer while stirring to make the gravy thicker. 5. Pour gravy over steaks and serve hot.

NUTRIENTS (PER SERVING):

Calories: 249 | Sodium: 128mg | Protein: 22g | Cholesterol: 149mg |
Potassium: 266mg | Carbs: 7g | Fiber: 1g

11. SWEDISH MEATBALLS

Servings: 35 meatballs   **Duration: 45 minutes**

INGREDIENTS	INSTRUCTIONS
• ¼ cup onions, finely chopped • 1 tsp Italian seasoning • 1 tbsp lemon juice • 1 pound lean ground beef • 1 tsp black pepper • ¼ tsp dry mustard • ¾ tsp onion powder • 1 tsp Tabasco® sauce • 1 tsp granulated sugar	1. Preheat the oven to 425°F. 2. Mix chopped onions, granulated sugar, beef, black pepper, onion powder, Italian seasoning, lemon juice, 1 tsp Tabasco® sauce, and dry mustard in a large bowl. 3. For each meatball, use 1 tbsp of the meat mixture. 4. Put the meatballs in a greased baking dish and bake for 20 minutes. 5. Take the meatballs out of the oven and mix with sauce. ***Serve on your favorite platter and enjoy.***

NUTRIENTS (PER SERVING):

Calories: 76 | Sodium: 31mg | Protein: 5g | Cholesterol: 21mg |
Potassium: 71mg | Carbs: 2g

12. TACO STUFFING

Servings: 8   **Duration: 45 minutes**

INGREDIENTS	INSTRUCTIONS
• 2 tbsp vegetable oil • ½ tsp ground red pepper • ½ head shredded lettuce • ½ tsp black pepper • 1 tsp garlic powder • 1 tsp onion powder • 1 tsp Italian seasoning • One medium taco shell • 1 ¼ pounds lean ground beef	1. Warm up oil. Mix onion powder, red pepper, Italian seasoning, black pepper, garlic powder and ground meat in a large skillet. 2. Cook until the beef is done, and all ingredients are mixed well. 3. Stuff 2 ounces of meat into taco shells and top with shredded lettuce. ***Serve your guest and enjoy your dinner with these meat wraps.***

NUTRIENTS (PER SERVING):

Calories: 176 | Sodium: 124mg | Protein: 14g | Cholesterol: 56g | Potassium: 258mg | Carbs: 9g

13. CLASSIC POT ROAST

Servings: 8   **Duration: 10 minutes to cook (5 hours to marinate)**

INGREDIENTS	INSTRUCTIONS
• ½ small, sweet onion, chopped • 1-pound boneless beef chuck • 1 tsp dried thyme • One cup plus 3 tbsp water • ½ tsp freshly ground black pepper • 1 tbsp olive oil • 2 tsp minced garlic • 2 tbsp cornstarch	1. Put a large stockpot over medium heat. 2. Add pepper to the roast. 3. Put the oil in the stockpot and brown all sides of the meat. 4. Put the meat on a plate and put it aside. 5. In a stockpot, sauté the onion and garlic for approximately 3 minutes or until softened. 6. Put the beef back in the pot with any collected juices, thyme, and 1 cup of water. 7. Bring the liquid to a boil, then turn down the heat so that it simmers. 8. Cover and let the beef simmer for about 4 1/2 hours or until it is very tender. 9. Mix the cornstarch and 3 tbsp of water together in a small bowl to make a slurry. 10. Whisk the slurry into the liquid in the pot, and then cook for 15 minutes to thicken the sauce.

NUTRIENTS (PER SERVING):

Calories: 159 | Fat: 10g | Carbohydrates: 2g | Phosphorus: 109mg | Potassium: 184mg | Sodium: 44mg | Protein: 14g

14. GRILLED MARINATED BEEF STEAKS

Servings: 6 **Duration: 30 minutes (5-6 hours marinating)**

INGREDIENTS	INSTRUCTIONS
• 1 ½ lb chuck steak • ¼ tsp pepper • ½ cup sliced green onion • 2 tbsp vinegar • 2 tbsp sugar • ¼ cup chopped green pepper • 2 cloves garlic, minced • 1 tbsp teriyaki sauce	1. Place the steak in a large shallow dish. Mix the rest of the ingredients together and pour over the steak. 2. Marinate in the fridge for 6 to 8 hours, turning at least once to let the flavors get in. Drain the steak and save the marinade. 3. Broil steak over medium coals for 15 to 20 minutes, coating with the marinade you stored. When perfectly cooked, let the steaks out for a broiler and *serve in your favorite platter and dressing.*

NUTRIENTS (PER SERVING):
Calories: 201 | Carbs: 12g | Protein: 25g | Fat: 6g | Sodium: 196mg |
Potassium: 484mg | Phosphorus: 247mg

15. PAN-FRIED PORK CHOP WITH CREAMY LEEK SAUCE

Servings: 2 **Duration: 30 minutes**

INGREDIENTS	INSTRUCTIONS
• 2 pork chops • 50ml milk • 1 garlic clove, peeled and chopped • 1 tbsp fresh parsley, chopped • 2 sprigs of thyme, leaves only • 1 tbsp vegetable oil • knob unsalted butter • ½ leek, washed and sliced • 150ml double cream	1. Heat the frying pan. Brush the pork chop with oil and put it in the pan to cook for six minutes. 2. Turn the chop over and cook for another 6 minutes or until it is browned and cooked through. 3. When perfectly cooked, the fluids will run clear when a sharp knife is inserted. Remove from heat and let it sit for three minutes. 4. For the leeks, heat the oil and butter in a pan. Add the leeks, thyme leaves, and garlic and cook for 3–4 minutes, until the leeks are soft. 5. Stir in milk, cream, and parsley, then reduce the heat and let it simmer for another 6–8 minutes while stirring continuously. *Serve the pork chop with the creamed leek sauce on top.*

NUTRIENTS (PER SERVING):
Calories: 343 | Carbs: 19g | Protein: 25g | Fat: 11g | Sodium: 196mg |
Potassium: 398mg | Phosphorus: 221mg

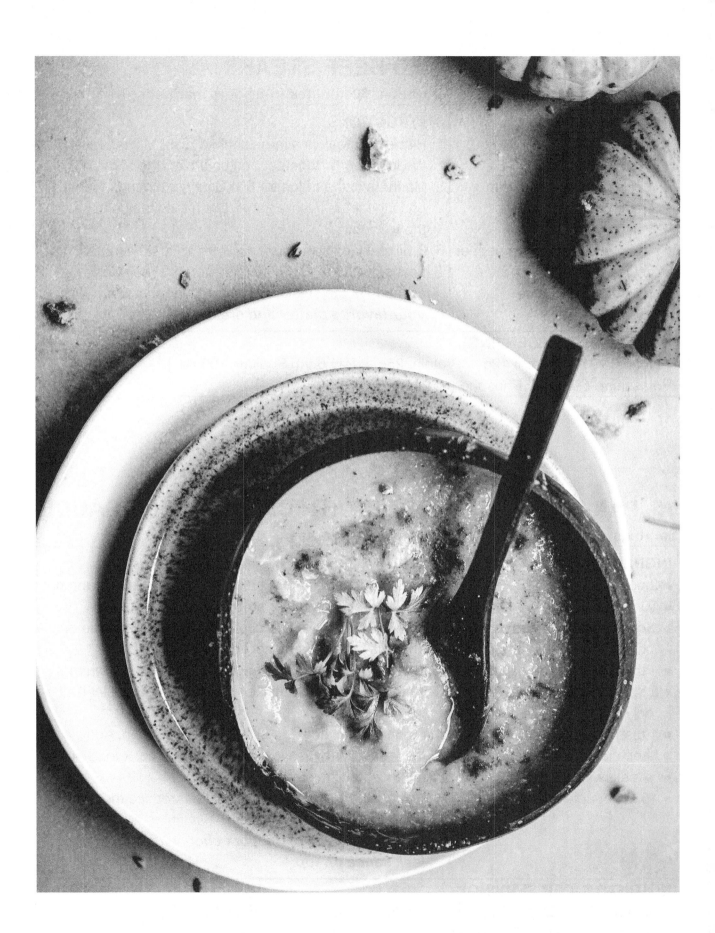

Chapter 12 SOUPS

1. Beans and Vegetables Soup

2. Paprika Pork Stew

3. Chicken Barley Soup

4. Spicy Chicken Soup

5. Beet Borscht

6. Herbed Cabbage Stew

7. Healthy Broccoli Soup

8. Traditional Chicken-Vegetable Soup

9. Chicken Noodle Soup

10. Curried Cauliflower Soup

11. Hearty Beef Veggie Soup

12. Lentil Tomato Soup

13. Spinach White Bean Soup

14. Best Curried Pumpkin Soup

15. French Onion Soup

A BOWL OF SOUP IS LIKE A WARM HUG FROM THE INSIDE.

IN THIS CHAPTER, YOU WILL FIND A VARIETY OF KIDNEY-FRIENDLY SOUP RECIPES THAT ARE PERFECT FOR ANY MEAL OR OCCASION. FROM BEANS AND VEGETABLES SOUP TO HEARTY BEEF VEGGIE SOUP, THESE RECIPES ARE BOTH DELICIOUS AND EASY TO PREPARE. WARM UP WITH THESE FLAVORFUL SOUPS THAT ARE TAILORED TO MEET THE DIETARY RESTRICTIONS OF THOSE ON A RENAL DIET.

1. PAPRIKA PORK STEW

Servings: 8   **Duration: 5-6 hours**

INGREDIENTS	INSTRUCTIONS
• 1 (2 pounds) boneless pork shoulder roast, trimmed of excess fat and cut into 1-inch cubes • 3 Yukon Gold potatoes, cubed • 3 carrots, sliced • 2 tbsp brown sugar • 3 tbsp all-purpose flour • 2 tbsp Worcestershire sauce • 2 cloves garlic, minced • ½ tsp salt • 2 ½ tbsp ground paprika • 1 cup beef stock • 2 onions, sliced • ¾ cup tomato sauce • 1 tbsp dried oregano • ½ tsp dry mustard • ¼ cup cold water • ¼ tsp ground black pepper	1. place carrots, onions, potatoes, and garlic in the slow cooker. On top of the vegetables, put the pork. 2. Mix the beef stock, paprika, Worcestershire sauce, oregano, brown sugar, tomato sauce, mustard, salt, and pepper in a bowl. Stir to mix. 3. Cover and cook on low heat for 6 to 7 hours or until the pork is fork-tender. Skim off the fat and move the meat and vegetables to one side of the cooker. 4. In a small bowl, mix cold water and flour until smooth. Pour the mixture into the slow cooker and stir to combine with the other ingredients. 5. Cover and cook on High for 10 to 15 minutes or until the sauce has thickened.

NUTRIENTS (PER SERVING):
Calories: 231 | Fat: 19g | Carbs: 18g | Protein: 12g | Cholesterol: 65mg | Fiber 3g

2. BEANS AND VEGETABLES SOUP

Servings: 4   **Duration: 45 minutes**

INGREDIENTS	INSTRUCTIONS
• 1 small onion, chopped • 5 cups chicken —stock • 2 medium potatoes diced • ¼ tsp dry basil • 1 medium chopped carrot • 2 cloves garlic chopped • 2 cups diced tomatoes • 3 cups green beans —cut into pieces • ½ tsp black pepper • 2 tbsp olive oil • 1 tsp salt	1. In a large saucepan, cook carrots and onion in olive oil for 3 minutes over medium heat. 2. Add the tomatoes, potatoes, chicken stock and garlic and bring to a boil. Add salt, pepper, and basil. 3. Reduce heat and let it cook for 15 minutes. Add green beans and simmer for 15 minutes more, until tender. 4. Simmer the soup for 15-20 minutes until all the vegetables are tender. Cooking time depends on the kind of pot, stove, vegetables, and amount of stock used. ***Garnish with chopped parsley or dill to the top and serve!***

NUTRIENTS (PER SERVING):

Calories: 335 | Fat: 17g | Cholesterol: 50mg | Sodium: 87mg | Carbs: 28g | Fiber: 7g | Sugar: 7g | Protein: 18g

3. CHICKEN BARLEY SOUP

Servings: 5   **Duration: 35 minutes**

INGREDIENTS	INSTRUCTIONS
• 8 cups water • 1-1/2 cups chopped carrots • ½ tsp poultry seasoning • 1 cup chopped celery • 1 bay leaf • ½ cup chopped onion • ½ tsp rubbed sage • 1 broiler/fryer chicken (2 to 3 pounds) • ½ cup medium pearl barley • 1 tsp chicken bouillon granules • ½ tsp pepper • 1 tsp salt, optional	1. Boil chicken in water in a large stockpot until it is cooked through and tender. Cool the broth and remove the fat and bone. Cut the meat into cubes. 2. Add the rest of the ingredients to the pan with the meat. Get it to boil. 3. Reduce the heat, cover, and let the soup cook for an hour or until the vegetables and barley are soft. Discard the bay leaf. ***Serve in your favorite soup bowl. Serve hot!***

NUTRIENTS (PER SERVING):

Calories: 151 | Fat: 5g | Carbs: 6g | Cholesterol: 89mg | Sodium: 22mg | Protein: 21g

4. SPICY CHICKEN SOUP

Servings: 4   **Duration: 40 minutes**

INGREDIENTS	INSTRUCTIONS
• 1 1"-piece ginger, peeled, chopped • 8 cups of low-sodium chicken broth • 2 garlic cloves, finely chopped • ½ tsp cayenne pepper • 1 tbsp olive oil • 2 cups baby spinach • 1 prepared rotisserie chicken • Kosher salt, freshly ground pepper • ½ cup sliced shiitake mushrooms • 2 scallions, thinly sliced • 1 medium onion, thinly sliced • Lime wedges (for serving)	1. Shred chicken meat and place it in a small bowl. Remove and discard the skin and bones. 2. In a large saucepan, heat the oil over medium-high heat. Add the onion and mushrooms and cook, stirring every so often, for 8–10 minutes, until the onion and mushrooms are soft and golden. 3. Add the garlic and ginger and cook for 2 minutes, stirring often. Season with salt and pepper to taste. Put the chicken shreds, broth, and cayenne pepper in the pot and bring to a boil. 4. Add the spinach, and then pour the soup into bowls. 5. Top with scallions and serve lime wedges alongside for squeezing over.

NUTRIENTS (PER SERVING):

Calories: 270 | Fat: 12g | Cholesterol: 192mg | Sodium: 287mg | Carbs: 10g |
Fiber: 2g | Protein: 16g

5. BEET BORSCHT

Servings: 8   **Duration: 45 minutes**

INGREDIENTS	INSTRUCTIONS
• 2 cups shredded fresh • 1 cup shredded cabbage beets • 1 cup shredded carrots • 2 cans (14-1/2 ounces each) beef broth • 1 cup chopped onion • 1 tbsp butter • 1/2 tsp salt • 2 cups water • Sour cream and chopped chives • 1 tbsp lemon juice	1. Bring the beets, carrots, onion, water, and salt to a boil in a saucepan. Turn down the heat, cover it, and let it cook for 20 minutes. 2. Add the broth, cabbage, and butter, and cook for 15 minutes with the lid off. Add lemon juice right before you serve. 3. Garnish with sour cream and chives or dill on top of each serving.

NUTRIENTS (PER SERVING):

Calories: 48 | Fat: 2g | Carbs: 17g | Cholesterol: 4mg | Sodium: 301mg | Protein: 2g

6. HERBED CABBAGE STEW

Servings: 6 **Duration: 35 minutes**

INGREDIENTS	INSTRUCTIONS
• 1 cup fresh green beans, cut into 1-inch pieces • 2 tbsp chopped fresh parsley • 3 celery stalks, chopped with the leafy tops • 1 tsp chopped savory • 1 tsp unsalted butter • 6 cups shredded green cabbage • ½ large, sweet onion, chopped • 1 tbsp chopped fresh thyme • 2 tbsp freshly squeezed lemon juice • 1 tsp minced garlic • 1 tsp chopped fresh oregano • Water • 1 scallion, chopped • Freshly ground black pepper	1. Melt the butter in a medium saucepan over medium-high heat. 2. For about 3 minutes, or until the onion and garlic are soft, sauté them in the melted butter. 3. Add the savory, celery, lemon juice, scallion, cabbage, parsley, thyme, and oregano to the pot. Then, add enough water to cover the vegetables by about 4 inches. 4. Bring the soup to a boil, reduce the flame, and let it simmer for about 25 minutes or until the vegetables are soft. 5. Put the green beans in and let them cook for 3 minutes. Add pepper to taste.

NUTRIENTS (PER SERVING):
Calories: 33 | Fat: 1g | Carbs: 6g | Phosphorus: 29mg | Potassium: 187mg | Sodium: 20mg | Protein: 1g

7. HEALTHY BROCCOLI SOUP

Servings: 4 **Duration: 30 minutes**

INGREDIENTS	INSTRUCTIONS
• ½ cup chopped onion • 1 can (12 ounces) fat-free evaporated milk • 2 cups chopped fresh broccoli • Olive oil, cracked black pepper (optional) • 1 can (14-1/2 ounces) reduced-sodium chicken broth • 2 tbsp cornstarch	1. In a large pot, combine the broccoli, onion, and broth. Simmer for 10 to 15 minutes or until the vegetables are soft. Blend half of the mixture in a blender, then put it back in the pot. 2. Mix 3 tbsp of milk and the corn flour in a small bowl until smooth. 3. Gradually add the remaining milk. Mix it in with the broccoli. Bring to a boil, then cook and stir for 2 minutes until the mixture thickens. Serve with a drizzle of olive oil and black pepper, if desired.

NUTRIENTS (PER SERVING):
Calories: 120 | |Fat: 0g | Carbs: 14g | Cholesterol: 4mg | Sodium: 20mg | Protein: 10g

8. TRADITIONAL CHICKEN-VEGETABLE SOUP

Servings: 6   **Duration: 35 minutes**

INGREDIENTS	INSTRUCTIONS
• 1 tbsp unsalted butter • Freshly ground black pepper • 2 cups chopped cooked chicken breast • 1 cup Easy Chicken Stock • 1 carrot, diced • 4 cups water • 2 tsp minced garlic • 1 tsp chopped fresh thyme • ½ sweet onion, diced • 2 tbsp chopped fresh parsley • 2 celery stalks, chopped	1. Melt the butter in a large pot over medium heat. 2. Heat the olive oil over medium heat in a skillet and sauté the onion and garlic until tender, about 3 minutes. Put in the chicken, celery, carrot, chicken stock, and water. 3. Bring the soup to a boil, reduce the heat, and let it simmer for about 30 minutes. 4. Stir in the thyme and let the soup simmer for 2 minutes. 5. Season with pepper and serve topped with parsley

NUTRIENTS (PER SERVING):
Calories: 121 | Fat: 6g | Carbs: 2g | Phosphorus: 108mg | Potassium: 199mg | Sodium: 62mg | Protein: 15g

9. CHICKEN NOODLE SOUP

Servings: 6   **Duration: 30 minutes**

INGREDIENTS	INSTRUCTIONS
• 1 tsp red pepper • ½ cup green pepper • 1 pound chicken parts • 1 tsp garlic powder • 1 tsp sugar • ½ cup celery • 1 tsp caraway seed • 1 tsp onion powder • 1 tsp oregano • 2 tbsp vegetable oil • ¼ cup lemon juice • 1 cup egg noodles • 3 ½ cups water • 1 tsp black pepper • 1 tbsp poultry seasoning	1. Brush chicken pieces with lemon juice. 2. Mix the chicken, water, garlic powder, caraway seed, onion powder, sugar, vegetable oil, red pepper, poultry seasoning, oregano, and black pepper in a large pot. 3. Cook the chicken for 30 minutes or until it is smooth. 4. Add the rest of the ingredients and cook for 15 minutes more. Prepare hot.

NUTRIENTS (PER SERVING):
Calories: 110 | Sodium: 17mg | Protein: 3g | Cholesterol: 12mg | Potassium: 102mg | Fat: 8g | Carbs: 7g | Phosphorus: 39mg | Fiber: 0g

10. CURRIED CAULIFLOWER SOUP

Servings: 6   **Duration: 30 minutes**

INGREDIENTS	INSTRUCTIONS
• 1 small, sweet onion, chopped • 3 cups water, or more to cover the cauliflower • 2 tsp curry powder • 1 tsp unsalted butter • ½ cup light sour cream • 1 small head cauliflower, cut into small florets • 3 tbsp chopped fresh cilantro • 2 tsp minced garlic	1. In a large frying pan, melt the butter over medium-high heat. Add the onion and garlic and cook for about 3 minutes until the onion and garlic are soft. 2. Mix in the cauliflower, water, and curry powder. 3. Bring the soup to a boil, reduce the flame and let it simmer for about 20 minutes or until the cauliflower is soft. 4. Pour the soup into a blender or food processor and blend it until it is smooth and creamy. 5. Put the soup back in the pot and add the sour cream and cilantro. 6. On medium-low, heat the soup for about 5 minutes or until warm. ***Drizzle some fresh cream on top and cilantro leaves.***

NUTRIENTS (PER SERVING):
Calories: 33 | Fat: 2g | Carbs: 4g | Phosphorus: 30mg | Potassium: 167mg | Sodium: 22mg | Protein: 1g

11. HEARTY BEEF VEGGIE SOUP

Servings: 9   **Duration: 3 hours**

INGREDIENTS	INSTRUCTIONS
• 1-pound lean ground beef (90% lean) • 1 package (10 ounces) frozen corn • 1 medium onion, chopped • 2 cups coleslaw mix • 2 tbsp Worcestershire sauce • 4 cups spicy hot V8 juice • 2 garlic cloves, minced • 1 tsp dried basil • 1 package (9 ounces) frozen cut green beans • 1 can (14-1/2 ounces) Italian stewed tomatoes • ¼ tsp pepper	1. Cook the beef and onion over medium heat in a large nonstick skillet until the meat is no longer pink. 2. Stir in garlic and cook for another minute. Drain. 3. Move to a slow cooker that holds 5 quarts. Mix in tomatoes, Worcestershire sauce, V8 juice, basil, coleslaw, and pepper. 4. Cover and cook on low for 3 to 4 hours or until heated through. Add the corn and green beans during the last 30 minutes of cooking. Serve immediately!

NUTRIENTS (PER SERVING):
Calories: 162 | Fat: 4g | Carbs: 18g | Cholesterol: 31mg | Sodium: 330mg | Protein: 13g

12. LENTIL TOMATO SOUP

Servings: 6   **Duration: 45 minutes**

INGREDIENTS	INSTRUCTIONS
• 1 medium onion, chopped • ½ tsp dried thyme • ⅔ cup dried brown lentils, rinsed • 1 tsp black pepper • 1 tbsp brown sugar • 2 tbsp minced fresh parsley • 1 tbsp white vinegar • 4 medium carrots, sliced • ¼ tsp dried tarragon • 1 tsp garlic salt • ¼ tsp dill weed • 1 can (6 ounces) tomato paste • 4-1/2 cups water	1. Put the water, carrots, onion, and lentils in a large saucepan and bring to a boil. 2. Reduce heat, cover, and let the food simmer for 20-25 minutes or until the lentils and vegetables are tender. Mix in the rest of the ingredients and boil it back again. 3. Lower the heat and let it simmer for 5 minutes to let the flavors mix.

NUTRIENTS (PER SERVING):

Calories: 138 | Protein: 8g | Cholesterol: 0mg | Potassium: 102mg | Fat: 0g | Carbs: 20g | Phosphorus: 39mg | Fiber: 9g | Sodium: 251mg

13. SPINACH WHITE BEAN SOUP

Servings: 8   **Duration: 6-7 hours**

INGREDIENTS	INSTRUCTIONS
• 2 garlic cloves, minced • 6 cups reduced-sodium vegetable broth • ½ cup rice, uncooked • 1 can (15-1/2 ounces) great northern beans, rinsed and drained • 1 tsp dried basil • 1/8 tsp salt • 1 can (15 ounces) tomato puree • ¼ cup shredded Parmesan cheese • ½ cup onion, chopped • 7 cups chopped fresh spinach • ¼ tsp pepper	1. Put the first 9 ingredients into a slow cooker that holds 4 quarts. 2. Cover and cook on low for 6 to 7 hours or until heated through. Stir in spinach. 3. Cover and cook for 15 minutes or until the spinach has wilted. ***Put cheese on top.***

NUTRIENTS (PER SERVING):

Calories: 151 | Fat: 1g | Carbs: 19g | Cholesterol: 20mg | Sodium: 230mg | Protein: 7g

14. BEST CURRIED PUMPKIN SOUP

Servings: 7   **Duration: 20 minutes**

INGREDIENTS	INSTRUCTIONS
• ¼ tsp ground nutmeg • ½ to 1 tsp curry powder • 1 can (15 ounces) pumpkin • ½ cup chopped onion • 1 can (12 ounces) evaporated milk • 2 tbsp all-purpose flour • 1 tbsp honey • 2 tbsp butter • ½ tsp salt • ½ to 1 tsp curry powder • ¼ tsp pepper • ½ pound fresh mushrooms, sliced • Minced chives • 3 cups vegetable broth	1. In a large saucepan, sauté the mushrooms and onion in butter until softened. Add the flour and curry powder and stir until well mixed. 2. Add the broth slowly. Bring to a boil, then cook and stir for 2 minutes until thickened. Add the pumpkin, milk, honey, salt, pepper, and nutmeg, and cook until everything mix well. Add chives as a garnish.

NUTRIENTS (PER SERVING):

Calories: 155 | Fat: 7g | Carbs: 11g | Cholesterol: 26mg | Sodium: 18mg | Protein: 6g

15. FRENCH ONION SOUP

Servings: 4   **Duration: 50 minutes**

INGREDIENTS	INSTRUCTIONS
• 2 cups water • 4 Vidalia onions, sliced thin • 1 tbsp chopped fresh thyme • 2 cups Easy Chicken Stock • 2 tbsp unsalted butter • Freshly ground black pepper	1. Melt the butter in a large saucepan on medium heat. 2. Add the onions to the pan and cook them slowly, stirring them often for about 30 minutes or until they are caramelized and soft. 3. Put the chicken stock and water into the soup and bring it to a boil. 4. Reduce heat and let the soup cook for 15 minutes. 5. Stir in thyme and pepper to taste. Serve hot.

NUTRIENTS (PER SERVING):

Calories: 90 | Fat: 6g | Carbohydrates: 7g | Phosphorus: 22mg |
Potassium: 192mg | Sodium: 57mg | Protein: 2g

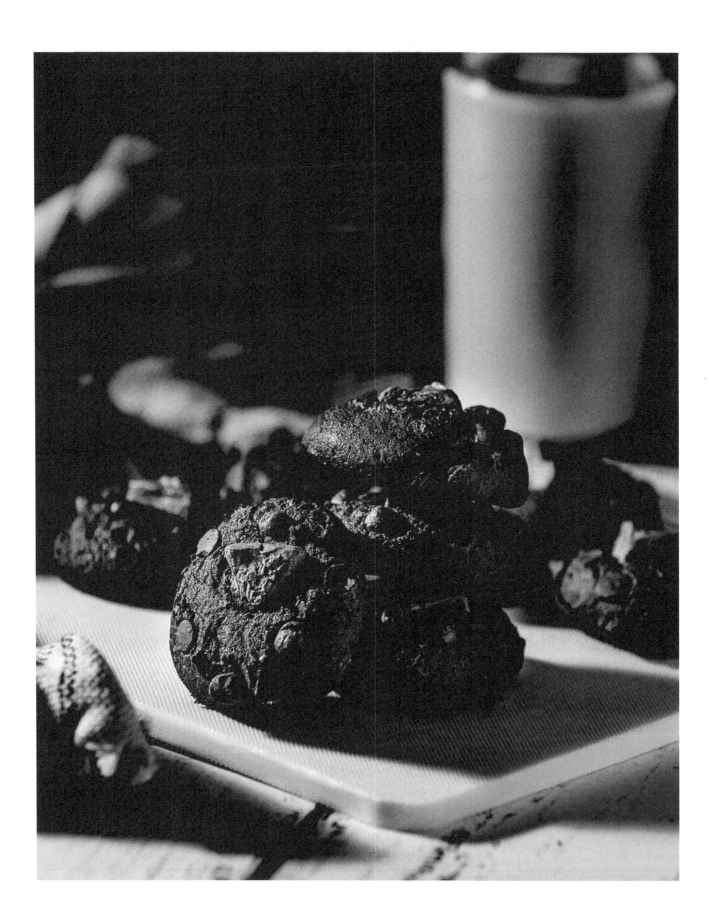

Chapter 13   SNACKS

1. Eggplant Chips

2. Roasted Asparagus with Pine Nuts

3. Cauliflower Snacks

4. Hummus with Celery

5. Mushroom Chips

6. Sweet and Spicy Kettle Corn

7. Blueberries and Cream Ice Pops

8. Cucumber-Wrapped Vegetable Rolls

9. Cheese-Herb Dip

10. Five-Spice Chicken Lettuce Wraps

11. Snack Mix

12. Spiced Pineapple Appetizer

13. Oriental Egg Rolls

14. Onion Bagel Chips

15. Chili Wheat Treats

SNACK TIME IS HAPPY TIME. ☺

IN THIS CHAPTER, YOU WILL FIND A VARIETY OF KIDNEY-FRIENDLY SNACK RECIPES THAT ARE PERFECT FOR SATISFYING THOSE MID-DAY CRAVINGS. FROM EGGPLANT CHIPS TO CHILI WHEAT TREATS THESE RECIPES ARE BOTH TASTY AND HEALTHY. LEARN HOW TO MAKE DELICIOUS SNACKS THAT MEET THE DIETARY RESTRICTIONS OF THOSE ON A RENAL DIET WITH THESE EASY-TO-FOLLOW RECIPES.

1. EGGPLANT CHIPS

Servings: 4　　　　　　　　**Duration: 30 minutes**

INGREDIENTS	INSTRUCTIONS
• ¼ tsp black pepper • 2 Japanese eggplants 1 lb. total weight, unpeeled • ½ tsp garlic powder • Olive oil spray • ½ tsp Diamond Crystal kosher salt	1. Slice the eggplant and put it in a large bowl. 2. Add the olive oil and spices to the bowl, and then gently toss the eggplant with tongs until each piece is covered in spices. 3. Put the eggplant slices on the trays of a drier and use the setting for fruits/vegetables (about 135 degrees) to dry them out for about 4 to 5 hours or until completely dry and crisp. 4. Check the trays in about 3–4 hours, as some thinner slices may be done before that. 5. Do not put eggplant in a container until it is completely cool.

NUTRIENTS (PER SERVING):
Calories: 420 | Carbs: 75g | Cholesterol: 0mg | Sodium: 83mg | Fiber: 22g | Sugar: 27g | Protein: 7g

2. ROASTED ASPARAGUS WITH PINE NUTS

Servings: 4   **Duration: 20 minutes**

INGREDIENTS	INSTRUCTIONS
• 2 pounds asparagus, trimmed, washed • ¼ cup parmesan • ½ tsp ground black pepper • 2 tbsp olive oil • ¼ cup pine nuts • parsley, chopped for garnish • ½ tsp salt	1. Preheat the oven to 425°F. 2. Lay out the asparagus in a row on a baking sheet. 3. Pour the olive oil on top, then sprinkle the salt and black pepper. Coat the asparagus well and spread them out again. 4. After 5 minutes, roast. Take it out of the oven and sprinkle the pine nuts on top. 5. Roast for another 5 more minutes, then take it out of the oven again. ***Top with parsley and parmesan cheese. Serve!***

NUTRIENTS (PER SERVING):
Calories: 95 | Carbs: 5g | Protein: 4g | Fat: 7g | Cholesterol: 3mg | Sodium: 202mg

3. CAULIFLOWER SNACKS

Servings: 2   **Duration: 30 minutes**

INGREDIENTS	INSTRUCTIONS
• 8 ounces Cauliflower (broken into flowerets) • 1/8 tsp dried tarragon • 2 tbsp unsalted butte • 1/8 tsp salt • 1/8 tsp dried marjoram • fresh black pepper (to taste)	1. Place an oven-proof pan at 325°F. When the pan is hot, spray it lightly with oil and add the cauliflower. 2. Put the pan back in the oven, roast the cauliflower, and occasionally toss it for about 20 to 25 minutes. 3. While roasting, put the spread, tarragon, salt, marjoram and pepper in a large bowl. 4. Cauliflower browned and roasted, take it out of the oven and put it in a spread bowl. Toss and coat the cauliflower with spread. Serve Immediately!

NUTRIENTS (PER SERVING):
Calories: 76 | Fat: 5g | Carbs: 6g | Sodium: 266mg | Protein: 3g

4. HUMMUS WITH CELERY

Servings: 8   **Duration: 20 minutes**

INGREDIENTS	INSTRUCTIONS
• 2 cans low sodium garbanzo beans • ¼ tsp salt • 3 cloves garlic • 4 tbsp lemons juiced • ½ cup tahini • 8 celery sticks	1. Pour 1/4 of the liquid from each of the two cans of beans. Put the beans and the rest of the liquid into the food processor. 2. Add garlic and lemon juice to the food processor. Blend the mixture until it is smooth and creamy. 3. Add tahini and salt. Blend until the mixture is smooth and creamy. ***Spread the hummus over celery sticks. Serve!***

NUTRIENTS (PER SERVING):
Calories: 127 | Fat: 6g | Carbs: 9g | Phosphorus: 85mg | Potassium: 118mg | Sodium: 64mg | Protein: 5g

5. MUSHROOM CHIPS

Servings: 2   **Duration: 1 hour**

INGREDIENTS	INSTRUCTIONS
• 8 oz. (230g) large button mushrooms • ¼ cup (60 ml) raw apple cider vinegar • ¼ cup (60 ml) extra-virgin olive oil • ½ tsp (or to taste) unrefined sea salt	1. Set the oven to 300°F. 2. Put parchment paper on a baking sheet. 3. Slice the mushrooms as thinly as you can. 4. Put the slices in a large bowl. 5. Pour the vinegar into it. Mix the vinegar to cover all of the mushroom slices. 6. Layer the mushroom slices on the baking sheet with parchment paper. 7. Now brush a lot of oil on both sides of the slices. Add salt to your taste. 8. Bake for approximately 45 minutes or until crispy and golden brown. Do not let it burn! 9. Let it cool to room temperature, remove the baking sheet, and serve.

NUTRIENTS (PER SERVING):
Fat: 6g | Carbs: 9g | Phosphorus: 82mg | Potassium: 118mg | Sodium: 90mg | Protein: 5g

6. SWEET AND SPICY KETTLE CORN

Servings: 6   **Duration: 10 minutes**

INGREDIENTS	INSTRUCTIONS
• 3 tbsp olive oil • Pinch cayenne pepper • ½ cup brown sugar • 1 cup popcorn kernels	1. Put a large pot with a lid over medium heat; add 3 tbsp olive oil and a few popcorn kernels. 2. Lightly shake the pot until the popcorn pops. Add the sugar and the rest of the corn kernels to the pot. 3. Pop the kernels by putting the lid on the pot and shaking it constantly until all kernels have popped. 4. Turn off the flame and pour the popcorn into a large bowl. ***Serve by Mixing the cayenne pepper with the popcorn.***

NUTRIENTS (PER SERVING):

Calories: 186 | Fat: 6g | Carbs: 30g | Phosphorus: 85mg | Potassium: 90mg | Sodium: 5mg | Protein: 3g

7. BLUEBERRIES AND CREAM ICE POPS

Servings: 6 pops   **Duration: 10 minutes (3 hours to marinate)**

INGREDIENTS	INSTRUCTIONS
• 1 tsp freshly squeezed lemon juice • ¼ tsp ground cinnamon • ¼ cup granulated sugar • ¼ cup light sour cream • 3 cups fresh blueberries • ¼ cup unsweetened rice milk • ½ tsp pure vanilla extract	1. Put the blueberries, lemon juice, vanilla, sour cream, rice milk, sugar, and cinnamon in a blender and blend until smooth. 2. Pour the mixture into ice-pop molds and freeze for 3 to 4 hours or until very firm.

NUTRIENTS (PER SERVING):

Calories: 78 | Fat: 1g | Carbs: 18g | Phosphorus: 20mg | Potassium: 55mg | Sodium: 12mg | Protein: 1g

8. CUCUMBER-WRAPPED VEGETABLE ROLLS

Servings: 8   **Duration: 30 minutes**

INGREDIENTS
- 1 English cucumber, sliced into 8 thin strips
- ½ cup finely shredded red cabbage
- ¼ cup chopped cilantro
- ¼ tsp freshly ground black pepper
- ½ cup grated carrot
- 1 tbsp olive oil
- ¼ cup julienned scallion, both green and white parts
- ¼ tsp ground cumin
- ¼ cup julienned red bell pepper

INSTRUCTIONS
1. Mix the cabbage, red pepper, carrot, scallion, olive oil, cilantro, cumin, and black pepper in a large bowl. Mix and combine well.
2. Spread the vegetable filling evenly on the cucumber strips and put it near one end of each strip.
3. Roll the cucumber strips around the filling and use a wooden pick to hold them together.
4. Repeat with each strip of cucumber.

NUTRIENTS (PER SERVING):
Calories: 26 | Fat: 2g | Carbs: 3g | Phosphorus: 14mg | Potassium: 95mg | Sodium: 7mg | Protein: 0g

9. CHEESE-HERB DIP

Servings: 8 (3 Tbsp. 1 serving) Duration: 20 minutes

INGREDIENTS
- ½ cup unsweetened rice milk
- 1 tsp minced garlic
- ½ scallion, green part, finely chopped
- 1 cup cream cheese
- 1 tbsp chopped fresh parsley
- 1 tbsp chopped fresh basil
- ½ tsp chopped fresh thyme
- 1 tbsp lemon juice
- ¼ tsp freshly ground black pepper

INSTRUCTIONS
1. Mix the cream cheese, lemon juice, milk, parsley, basil, thyme, scallion, garlic, and pepper in a medium bowl until well-mixed.
2. The dip can be kept in the fridge for up to a week in a sealed container.

NUTRIENTS (PER SERVING):
Calories: 108 | Fat: 10g | Carbs: 3g | Phosphorus: 40mg | Potassium: 52mg | Sodium: 112mg | Protein: 2g

10. FIVE-SPICE CHICKEN LETTUCE WRAPS

Servings: 8   **Duration: 30 minutes**

INGREDIENTS	INSTRUCTIONS
<ul><li>6 ounces cooked chicken breast, minced</li><li>2 tbsp chopped fresh cilantro</li><li>½ red apple, cored and chopped</li><li>¼ English cucumber, finely chopped</li><li>½ cup bean sprouts</li><li>Juice of 1 lime</li><li>1 scallion, both green and white parts, chopped</li><li>Zest of 1 lime</li></ul>	1. Mix the scallions, apple, chicken, cucumber, lime juice, bean sprouts, lime zest, cilantro, and five-spice powder together in a large bowl. 2. Put an equal amount of the chicken mixture on each of the 8 lettuce leaves. 3. Wrap the chicken mix in the lettuce and serve.

NUTRIENTS (PER SERVING):
Calories: 51 | Fat: 2g | Carbs: 2g | Phosphorus: 56mg | Potassium: 110mg | Sodium: 16mg | Protein: 7g

11. SNACK MIX

Servings: 6   **Duration: 20 minutes**

INGREDIENTS	INSTRUCTIONS
<ul><li>1 cup rice cereal squares</li><li>1/3 cup margarine, melted</li><li>1 tbsp Parmesan cheese</li><li>1 cup unsalted tiny pretzel twists</li><li>½ tsp garlic powder</li><li>1 cup corn cereal squares</li><li>½ tsp onion powder</li><li>3 cups unsalted popped popcorn</li></ul>	1. In a large bowl, mix together cereal, pretzels, and popcorn. Mix garlic powder and onion powder with melted margarine. 2. Pour the mixture over the cereal and toss to coat. Put in some Parmesan. 3. Bake in 350°F oven for 7–10 minutes. Cool. Store in an air-tight container.

NUTRIENTS (PER SERVING):
Calories: 180 | Carbs: 19g | Protein: 2.5g | Fat: 11g | Sodium: 386mg | Potassium: 37mg | Phosphorus: 38mg

12. SPICED PINEAPPLE APPETIZER

Servings: 10 (5 pieces per serving)   Duration: 20 minutes

INGREDIENTS	INSTRUCTIONS
• 1 20-oz can pineapple chunks in juice, drained • ½ tsp Dijon mustard • ¼ cup white vinegar • 2 tbsp lime juice • 1/8 tsp garlic powder • ¼ tsp crushed red pepper • 3 tbsp sugar	1. Mix the vinegar, sugar, lime juice, Dijon mustard, pepper, and garlic powder in a saucepan. Bring to a boil. 2. Reduce the flame and let it cook for 3 minutes, uncovered. 3. Mix the vinegar mixture and the pineapple together in a bowl. Serve Warm with toothpicks.

NUTRIENTS (PER SERVING):

Calories: 47 | Carbs: 12g | Protein: 0g | Fat: 0g | Sodium: 4mg |
Potassium: 67mg | Phosphorus: 4mg

13. ORIENTAL EGG ROLLS

Servings: 14   Duration: 20 minutes

INGREDIENTS	INSTRUCTIONS
• 1 lb. diced cooked chicken • 2 tbsp vegetable oil • ½ lb. bean sprouts • 1 tbsp low sodium soy sauce • 1 medium chopped onion • 1 clove garlic, minced • 1 package (20) egg roll wrappers • 1/2 lb shredded cabbage • Oil for frying	1. In a bowl, mix garlic, shredded cabbage, soy sauce, beans, onion and diced chicken together except the wrappers and the oil for frying. Let it marinate for 30 minutes. 2. Divide the filling between the wrappers and fold them as it says on the package. Warm the oil up. 3. Fry egg rolls in 1 inch or more of hot oil until golden brown. Drain onto paper towels.

NUTRIENTS (PER SERVING):

Calories: 168 | Carbs: 15g | Protein: 9g | Fat: 8g | Sodium: 152mg |
Potassium: 114mg | Phosphorus: 76mg

14. ONION BAGEL CHIPS

Servings: 4   **Duration: 20 minutes**

INGREDIENTS	INSTRUCTIONS
• 2 tbs margarine, melted • 2 3 1/2 –oz. plain bagels • 1/2 tsp onion powder	1. Use an electric knife to cut each bagel in half down the middle. Cut 8 vertical slices from one bagel half, cut side down, on a level surface. Repeat with the other halves of the bagels. 2. Place slices on a baking sheet. Mix margarine and onion powder together and spread on the bagels. 3. Bake for 20 minutes at 325°F or until golden brown and crisp. Exclude from pan and let cool completely. ***Put it in a container that will not let air in.***

NUTRIENTS (PER SERVING):

Calories: 128 | Carbs: 16g | Protein: 3g | Fat: 6g | Sodium: 208mg |
Potassium: 24mg | Phosphorus: 24mg

15. CHILI WHEAT TREATS

Servings: 8   **Duration: 20 minutes**

INGREDIENTS	INSTRUCTIONS
• ½ cup margarine • ½ tsp ground cumin • 4 cups spoon-size shredded wheat • Dash cayenne pepper • 1 tbsp chili powder • ½ tsp garlic powder	1. Turn oven on to 300°F. In a 10x15-inch baking pan, melt the margarine. Add spices and stir. 2. Add the cereal and stir well to coat it evenly. Bake for 15 minutes, until crispy. 3. When done, cut it into a square shape and keep it in an air-tight container. ***Serve a snack with any herb dip and enjoy!***

NUTRIENTS (PER SERVING):

Calories: 184 | Carbs: 16g | Protein: 3g | Fat: 12g | Sodium: 107mg |
Potassium: 104mg | Phosphorus: 82mg

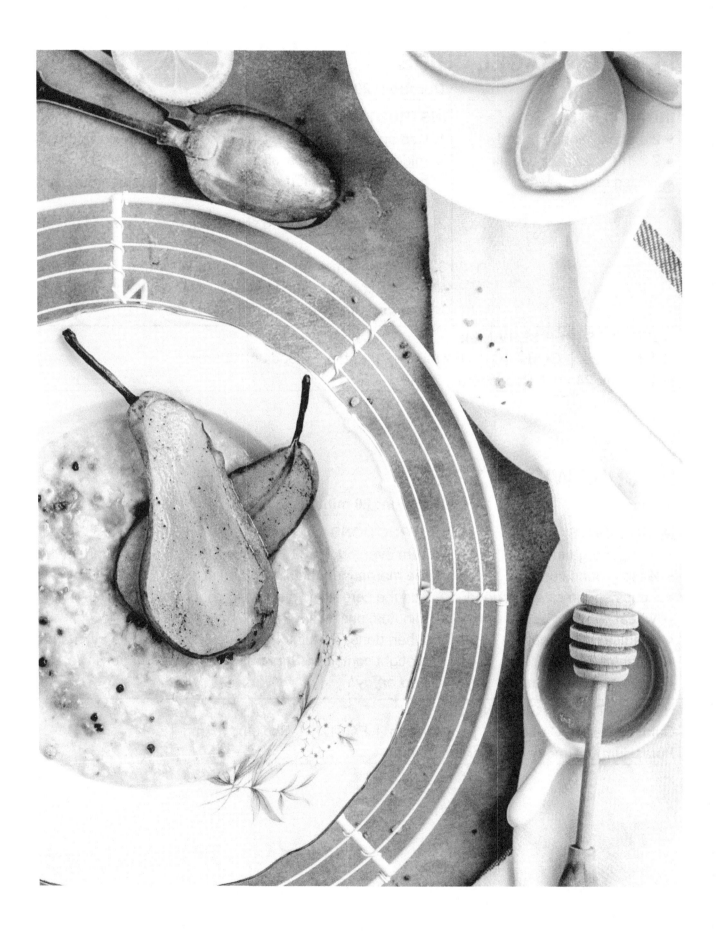

Chapter 14   DESSERTS

1. Chocolate Muffins

2. Strawberry Tiramisu

3. Pine-Apple Fruit Whip

4. Lemon Cake

5. Frozen Lemon Dessert

6. Chinese Almond Cookies

7. Cinnamon Crispies

8. Peanut Butter Swirl Fudge

9. Five Minutes Nutella Mug Cake

10. Hot Fruit Compote

11. Maple Crisp Bars

12. Chocolate Chip Cookies (Sugar-Free)

13. Brandy Apple Crisp

14. Cream Cheese Cookies

15. Fruity Rice Pudding

LIFE IS UNCERTAIN, BUT DESSERT DOES NOT HAVE TO BE!

IN THIS CHAPTER, YOU WILL FIND A VARIETY OF KIDNEY-FRIENDLY DESSERT RECIPES THAT ARE PERFECT FOR THOSE WITH A SWEET TOOTH. FROM CHOCOLATE MUFFINS TO FRUITY RICE PUDDING, THESE RECIPES ARE BOTH DELICIOUS AND HEALTHY. LEARN HOW TO MAKE SATISFYING DESSERTS THAT MEET THE DIETARY RESTRICTIONS OF THOSE ON A RENAL DIET WITH THESE EASY-TO-FOLLOW RECIPES.

1. CHOCOLATE MUFFINS

Servings: 12 **Duration: 45 minutes**

INGREDIENTS	INSTRUCTIONS
• 1 large egg • ½ cup milk • ½ cup unsweetened cocoa powder • 1 tsp baking powder • 1 cup fat-free yogurt • 2 cups all-purpose flour • ½ cup vegetable oil • 1 cup semisweet chocolate chips, divided • 1 tsp vanilla extract • ½ cup sugar or (stevia extract)	1. Set the oven's temperature to 400°F. Use paper muffin liners to line 12 muffin cups. 2. Mix the flour, sugar, 3/4 cup chocolate chips, cocoa powder, and baking soda in a large bowl. 3. Whisk yogurt, milk, oil, egg, vanilla, and vanilla extract in separate bowls until smooth. Pour the yogurt mixture into the chocolate mixture and stir until the batter is mixed. 4. Fill muffin tins 3/4 of the way and sprinkle the last 1/4 cup of chocolate chips on top. 5. Bake in an oven that has already been heated for about 20 minutes or until a toothpick stuck in the middle comes out clean. After 10 minutes, remove from pans and cool on wire racks. Store it in a fridge to maintain its freshness. ***Serve and enjoy with your favorite chocolate smoothie.***

NUTRIENTS:

Calories: 322 | Carbs: 18g | Fat: 12g | Sodium: 132mg | Cholesterol: 18mg | Potassium: 198mg | Protein: 5g

2. STRAWBERRY TIRAMISU

Servings: 6   **Duration: 20 minutes**

INGREDIENTS	INSTRUCTIONS
• ⅓ cup strawberry jam • 1 cup mascarpone cheese • ½ cup confectioners' sugar • ¼ cup water • ½ cup heavy whipping cream • 2 cups sliced strawberries • 24 ladyfingers • ½ tsp balsamic vinegar • ½ tsp vanilla extract	1. Mix mascarpone cheese, cream, sugar, and vanilla extract in a small bowl. Beat for 1 to 1 ½ minutes on medium-high speed with an electric blender until smooth and thickened. 2. Mix the strawberry preserves, water, and balsamic vinegar with a fork. Mix everything with a fork. 3. Layer half of the sliced strawberries and half of the mascarpone mixture on top of the ladyfingers. 4. Repeat the process with the rest of the ladyfingers. 5. Wrap it in plastic wrap and put it in the fridge for at least 8 hours or overnight.

NUTRIENTS:
Calories: 406 | Carbs: 39g | Protein: 8g | Fat: 17g | Cholesterol: 162mg | Sodium: 100mg | Potassium: 153mg | Fiber: 2g

3. PINE-APPLE FRUIT WHIP

Servings: 8   **Duration: 30 minutes (2-3 hours in the freezer)**

INGREDIENTS	INSTRUCTIONS
• 2 tbsp honey • 1 cup canned unsweetened pineapple juice • 2 cups unsweetened applesauce • ¼ tsp grated lemon peel • 1 envelope of unflavored gelatin • Cinnamon or nutmeg	1. Sprinkle gelatin over pineapple juice and let it sit for a few minutes to soften and stir the mixture over low heat until the gelatin is dissolved. Add lemon peel, honey, and applesauce to the bowl. 2. Keep in the fridge and stir frequently. Beat until the mixture rises slightly when dropped from a spoon. Divide among 8 dessert dishes. Chill and serve. 3. Sprinkle some cinnamon or nutmeg on top of each one.

NUTRIENTS:
Calories: 71 | Carbs: 18g | Protein: 2g | Fat: 0g | Sodium: 3mg | Potassium: 114mg | Phosphorus: 8mg

4. LEMON CAKE

Servings: 8   **Duration: 1 hour**

INGREDIENTS

- 2 large eggs
- 1 ¾ tsp baking powder
- ¾ cup milk
- ½ cup butter
- 1 tbsp lemon zest
- ½ sugar
- 1 ½ cups all-purpose flour
- 2 tsp vanilla extract
- 1 tbsp lemon juice

INSTRUCTIONS

1. Preheat the oven to 350°F. Grease a square 9-inch baking dish.
2. Using an electric mixer, beat the sugar and butter to light and fluffy. Add the eggs and vanilla extract and beat until they are well mixed.
3. Sift the flour and baking powder together in a separate bowl, then stir them into the creamed mixture.
4. Pour the milk, lemon zest, and lemon juice into the bowl and stir until smooth.
5. Put batter into the pan that has been set up. Bake in a preheated oven for about 35 minutes until a toothpick stuck in the middle comes out clean.

NUTRIENTS:

Calories: 251 | Carbs: 31g | Sodium: 173mg | Cholesterol: 63mg | Protein: 4g | Vitamin C: 2mg

5. FROZEN LEMON DESSERT

Servings: 9   **Duration: 1 hour**

INGREDIENTS

- 1 tsp Lemon Flavor
- ¼ tsp Baking Soda
- 32 oz. plain, nonfat Greek yogurt
- 1 tsp Vanilla Extract
- 3 tbsp Organic Corn Starch
- 1 tsp Xanthan Gum
- 5 tbsp Homemade Limoncello
- 1 tsp Natural Butter Flavor
- ¼ tsp Salt
- 2 tsp Liquid Stevia Extract

INSTRUCTIONS

1. Add the yogurt, stevia, lemon flavor, vanilla extract, butter flavor, Limoncello and lemon extract into a blender. Mix until smooth.
2. Whisk the cornstarch, baking soda, xanthan gum and salt together in a small bowl. Slowly add the dry ingredients while the blender is running. Mix until it is smooth. *(For color, feel free to add yellow food color)*
3. Put the frozen ice cream maker attachment on the stand mixer and turn it to "stir" speed. Pour the ice cream mixture into the cake pan and churn it until it has a soft-serve consistency.
4. Place the ice cream in a freezer-safe dish. Cover and freeze it for 3-5 hours or until it is the texture you like. Serve and enjoy!

NUTRIENTS:

Calories: 130 | Carbs: 16g | Fat: 7g | Sodium: 75mg | Cholesterol: 56mg | Protein: 2g

6. CHINESE ALMOND COOKIES

Servings: 24 (3 cookies per serving)   Duration: 30 minutes

INGREDIENTS	INSTRUCTIONS
• 1 tsp almond extract • 1 cup margarine, softened • 3 cups flour • 1 tsp baking soda • ½ cup sugar (or stevia extract) • 1 egg	1. Mix the margarine and sugar in a medium bowl. Add egg and beat well. 2. Sift the dry ingredients and add them to the creamed mixture. Add almond extract and stir well. 3. Roll into balls that are about 3/4 of an inch across. Put a small hole in the middle of each biscuit by pressing it. Bake the cookies at 400°F for 10 to 12 minutes or until the edges are golden brown.

NUTRIENTS:

Calories: 158 | Carbs: 20g | Fat: 8g | Sodium: 99mg | Potassium: 18mg | Phosphorus: 17mg | Protein: 2g

7. CINNAMON CRISPIES

Servings: 4   Duration: 20 minutes

INGREDIENTS	INSTRUCTIONS
• 2 tbsp margarine, melted • ½ tsp vanilla • 1 tsp cinnamon • 1 tbsp hot water • 1 ½ tbsp sugar • 4 6-inch flour tortillas	1. In a small bowl, mix the water and vanilla well. Take another bowl and combine sugar and cinnamon; stir well. 2. Brush margarine on both sides of a tortilla, then brush each side with a mixture of water and sugar. 3. Place the tortillas on a wire rack in a jelly roll pan. Bake for 6-7 minutes at 400°F or until the top is lightly browned. ***Serve and store in your favorite jar.***

NUTRIENTS:

Calories: 168 | Carbs: 21g | Protein: 3g | Fat: 8g | Sodium: 83mg | Potassium: 35mg | Phosphorus: 26mg

8. PEANUT BUTTER SWIRL FUDGE

Servings: 20   **Duration: 2 hours**

INGREDIENTS	INSTRUCTIONS
• 20 ounces chocolate chips bags • 1 ½ tsp vanilla • 1 tbsp coconut oil • 1/4 cup coconut sugar • 1 cup peanut butter crunchy • 1 cup coconut milk canned (I recommend Native Forest) • pinch of salt	1. Stir together the chocolate, coconut milk, sugar, chips and salt in a heavy saucepan on medium heat. 2. Mix the chocolate chips and reduce heat until all melted. 3. Stir to mix in the vanilla and coconut oil. Spread fudge into an 8x8-inch pan lined with parchment paper. 4. Add peanut butter to the top and use a toothpick to swirl the peanut butter into the chocolate. Be careful not to swirl too much—just enough to get the swirling effect.

NUTRIENTS:

Calories: 214 | Carbs: 21g | Protein: 4g | Fat: 14g | Cholesterol: 4mg |
Sodium: 20mg | Fiber: 1g | Sugar: 18g

9. FIVE MINUTES NUTELLA MUG CAKE

Servings: 2   **Duration: 5 minutes**

INGREDIENTS	INSTRUCTIONS
• 3 tbsp cocoa powder (not drink mix) • 3 tbsp Nutella • 3 tbsp milk • 4 tbsp self-rising flour • 1 large free-range egg • 3 tbsp vegetable oil • 2 tbsp sugar	1. Whisk all the dry ingredients together. Put the same amount in each of the two mugs. Take another bowl and the remaining ingredients together until smooth. 2. Divide these between the two mugs so that each has an equal amount, and then whisk each one until smooth. 3. Each one needs 1 to 2 minutes in the microwave until it has risen and set. Just wait a few minutes before serving. ***Before serving, add whipped cream and chocolate sauce to the top and enjoy.***

NUTRIENTS:

Calories: 382 | Carbs: 32g | Fat: 12g | Sodium: 46mg | Cholesterol: 93mg | Protein: 6g

10. HOT FRUIT COMPOTE

Servings: 12   **Duration: 45 minutes**

INGREDIENTS	INSTRUCTIONS

• 2 cups crushed cornflakes
• **1 (28 oz) can each:**
  (Peach slices, juice packed)
  (Pineapple chunks, juice packed)
  (Pear slices, juice packed)
• ¼ cup margarine, melted
• Cherry pie filling
	1. Drain fruit. Grease a 9-by-13-inch pan and put fruit in layers, finishing with pie filling.
	2. Crush cornflakes, mix them with margarine, and sprinkle them over the fruit. Bake at 350°F for 30 minutes. Serve hot!

NUTRIENTS:

Calories: 213 | Carbs: 40g | Fat: 4g | Phosphorus: 32mg | Sodium: 115mg |
Protein: 1.5g

11. MAPLE CRISP BARS

Servings: 20   **Duration: 20 minutes**

INGREDIENTS	INSTRUCTIONS
• 1 cup sugar • 1/3 cup margarine • 1/2 cup maple pancake syrup • 1 tsp maple extract • 8 cups puffed rice cereal	1. Melt margarine over medium heat in a large saucepan. Add the sugar, extract, and syrup, and stir. Bring to a boil. Remove from heat. 2. Stir in cereal and coat it well with the sugar mixture. 3. Press into a 13-by-9-inch greased baking pan. Chill. Divide into 20 pieces.

NUTRIENTS:

Calories: 110 | Carbs: 21g | Protein: 0g | Fat: 3g | Sodium: 26mg |
Potassium: 10mg | Phosphorus: 6mg

12. CHOCOLATE CHIP COOKIES (SUGAR-FREE)

Servings: 18   **Duration: 20 minutes**

INGREDIENTS	INSTRUCTIONS
• ½ tsp baking soda • ½ cup semi-sweet chocolate chips • ½ tsp vanilla • ½ cup margarine or butter • 1 cup flour • 1 egg, beaten • 4 tsp liquid sugar substitute • ¼ tsp salt	1. Whisk the dry ingredients. Melt margarine in a pan over medium heat. Stir in sugar substitute, vanilla, and egg. Add the flour mixture and combine all the ingredients well. 2. Add chocolate chips and stir. 3. Drop by teaspoonfuls on a greased baking sheet. Bake for 10 minutes at 375°F. Check meanwhile. Let the cookies chill and Serve!

NUTRIENTS:

Calories: 99 | Carbs: 8g | Protein: 1.4g | Fat: 7g | Sodium: 98mg | Potassium: 28mg | Phosphorus: 19mg

13. BRANDY APPLE CRISP

Servings: 6   **Duration: 1 hour**

INGREDIENTS	INSTRUCTIONS
• 4 cups tart apples peeled and chopped • 2 tbsp sugar • 2 tsp lemon juice • ½ tsp cinnamon • 1/8 tsp nutmeg • 2 tbsp flour • 2 tbsp margarine • ¼ cup brown sugar • 3/4 cup dry oats	1. Mix the first six ingredients in a square 8-inch baking dish. Mix well, then set aside. 2. Mix oats, brown sugar, and flour in a small bowl. Melt the margarine in until it is well mixed. Drizzle over apple mixture. Bake at 350°F for 45 minutes. 3. Serve hot or chilled according to your taste.

NUTRIENTS:

Calories: 203 | Carbs: 29g | Protein: 2g | Fat: 5g | Sodium: 36mg | Potassium: 159mg | Phosphorus: 59mg

14. CREAM CHEESE COOKIES

Servings: 7   **Duration: 30 minutes**

INGREDIENTS	INSTRUCTIONS
• 1 tsp vanilla extract candied cherry halves • 1 cup butter or margarine, softened • 1 cup sugar • 1 3-ounce package cream cheese, softened • 1 egg yolk • 2½ cups all-purpose flour	1. Set the temperature of the oven to 325°F. 2. Mix the butter and cream cheese together, then slowly add the sugar while beating until the mixture is fluffy. 3. Beat egg yolk, then add flour and vanilla, and mix well. 4. Let the dough chill for at least an hour. 5. Roll 1" balls of dough on a greased baking sheet. 6. Press a cherry half into each cookie in a gentle way. 7. Bake for 12-15 minutes.

NUTRIENTS:

Calories: 80 | Fat: 4g | Cholesterol: 13mg | Protein: 0.5g | Carbs: 11g | Fiber: 0g | Sodium: 31mg | Potassium: 15mg | Phosphorus: 14mg

15. FRUITY RICE PUDDING

Servings: 6   **Duration: 40 minutes**

INGREDIENTS	INSTRUCTIONS
• 2 cups Cool Whip® Light Whipped Topping • 1 sachet sugar substitute • 1 cup water • cinnamon (optional) • 1 cup Minute® rice (uncooked) • 1 can (14 oz.) no sugar added pineapple	1. Mix pineapple with water. Microwave for 5 minutes on high. 2. Add Minute rice and sugar substitute in an oven-proof dish. Cover with foil and wait 30 minutes. 3. Now bake the rice pudding for 1 hour at 300°F. Add Cool Whip® Light Whipped Topping and mix well. Divide among 6 small bowls and drizzle with cinnamon (if desired). You can serve it with your favorite fruits, jam and jellies on top. Enjoy!

NUTRIENTS:

Calories: 220 | Fat: 14g | Cholesterol: 42mg | Protein: 11g | Carbs: 49g | Fiber: 6g | Sodium: 131mg | Potassium: 15mg

The "30-day meal plan" section includes recipes for breakfast, lunch, dinner, and snacks, ensuring that individuals are well-nourished throughout the day. The recipes are kidney-friendly and delicious, making the meal plan a sustainable and enjoyable way to follow a renal diet.

By incorporating these recipes into your renal diet plan, you are taking care of your health, exploring new flavors, and expanding your culinary skills. It is important to remember that a renal diet does not have to be bland - plenty of delicious and creative options are available that meet the dietary restrictions.

With the help of this RENAL DIET COOKBOOK FOR BEGINNERS, you can enjoy various kidney-friendly meals and snacks that are both satisfying and nutritious. So why not try out some of these recipes today and discover how tasty and enjoyable a renal diet can be?

Your body and taste buds will thank you!

30-DAYS MEAL PLAN
B = Breakfast, **L** = Lunch, **D** = Dinner, **S** = Snack

DAY 1

B	Reuben Sandwich
L	Fried Bean Rice
D	Spicy Chicken Wings

DAY 2

B	Herbed Omelet
L	Yellow Squash & Green Onions
D	Lamb Chops
S	Batty Bites

DAY 3

B	Lemon Poppy Seed Muffins
L	Bow-Tie Pasta Salad
D	Baked Tilapia Fish with Garlic Sauce

DAY 4

B	Blueberry-Pineapple Smoothie
L	Easy Fish Cakes
D	Leek, Potato, and Carrot Soup

DAY 5

B	Cheese Coconut Pancake
L	Chicken Wraps
D	Easy lentil soup
S	Crunchy Crunch

DAY 6

B	Zucchini Scramble
L	Baked Halibut
D	New Orleans-Style Red Beans and Rice

DAY 7

B	Fruit and Oat Pancakes
L	Swedish Meatballs
D	Grilled Corn on the Cob

DAY 8

B	Egg and Veggie Muffins
L	Taco stuffing
D	Chicken & Pasta Salad
S	Cheese Herb Dip

DAY 9

B	Whole-grain English Muffins
L	Pork Souvlaki
D	Golden Potato Croquettes

DAY 10

B	Curried Egg Pita Pockets
L	Steak Mango Salad
D	Apple Baked Pork Chops

DAY 11

B	Fruit Salad and Yoghurt
L	Beef stew
D	Chili Rice with Red Beans

DAY 12

B	Summer Grilled Veggie Sandwich
L	Eggs and Avocado Salad
D	Cilantro-Lime Flounder

DAY 13

B	High Energy Porridge
L	Hearty Tuna Salad
D	Grilled Marinated Beef Steaks

DAY 14

B	Mexican Brunch Egg
L	Leaf Lettuce and Asparagus Salad with Raspberries
D	Smoked Mackerel Paté
S	Spicy Kale Chips

DAY 15

B	Shrimp Bruschetta
L	Steamed Asparagus
D	Salmon Stuffed Pasta Shells

DAY 16

B	Homemade Granola
L	Pumpkin Risotto
D	Beef Broth

DAY 17

B	Mixed-Grain Hot Cereal
L	Broiled Maple Salmon Fillets
D	Renal-Safe Macaroni & cheese
S	Peach Crisp

DAY 18

B	Dutch Apple Pancakes
L	Peppercorn Pork Chops
D	Asian Green bean and veggie salad

DAY 19

B	Renal Friendly Bran Muffins
L	Stuffed Green Peppers
D	Chicken Soup with Star Anise

DAY 20

B	Low Phosphorus Pancakes
L	Summer Chickpea salad
D	Chicken Stew
S	Grilled Salsa

DAY 21

B	Corn Pudding
L	Spanish Rice with Roasted Cauliflower
D	Baja Fish tacos
S	Baba Ghanoush

DAY 22

B	Cinnamon-Nutmeg Blueberry Muffin
L	Sesame Cucumber Salad
D	Broiled Garlic Shrimp
S	Blueberry and Cream Ice Pops

DAY 23

B	Grilled Chicken Sandwich
L	Italian Turkey Salad
D	Tangy Beef & vegetable kabobs

DAY 24

B	Feta mint Omelet
L	Grilled Fish in Foil
D	Waldorf Salad

DAY 25

B	Watermelon-raspberry Smoothie
L	Vegetables & Fried Rice
D	Parmesan Baked Fish
	Seasoned Green Beans
S	Spicy Kale Chips

DAY 26

B	Apple-Chia Smoothie
L	Open-faced turkey burgers
D	Honey Garlic Chicken
S	Caramel Rolls

DAY 27

B	Pizza Omelet
L	Fruity zucchini salad
D	Pork with Bell Peppers

DAY 28

B	Skillet Baked Pancake
L	Open-Faced Beef Stir-Up
D	Chicken Tortellini soup Bowl
S	Antojitos

DAY 29

B	Egg and Veggie Muffins
L	Onion Smothered Steak
D	Stewed Pigeon Peas
S	Cucumber-wrapped Vegetable Rolls

DAY 30

B	French Toast
L	Salmon in Dill sauce
D	Vegetarian Curry

CONCLUSION

In conclusion, the RENAL DIET COOKBOOK is an essential guide for individuals with renal disease who want to manage their condition through diet and exercise. The book provides comprehensive information on renal disease, including its causes, symptoms, and stages, as well as the benefits of the renal diet and guidelines for meal planning and preparation. The book also includes information on the nutrients that need to be regulated in the renal diet and a list of foods to avoid.

A healthy renal diet is not just about restriction; it is about nourishing our bodies and supporting our kidney health. The recipes in the cookbook are typically low in sodium, potassium, and phosphorus, and are tailored to meet the nutritional needs of people with kidney disease. We prioritize our kidney health and make dietary decisions keeping that goal in mind. In addition to the valuable information and practical tips provided in this book, we have included various delicious and healthy recipes specifically designed for those with renal disease.

We encourage you to try our recipes and make healthy eating a part of your daily routine. Implementing dietary guidelines can aid in weight loss and enhance your health, such as blood pressure regulation, and heart health. Overall, the renal diet cookbook aims to support people with kidney disease in making healthy food choices that can help to improve their overall health and well-being.

Our kidneys may be small, but they have a big job. With the proper care and support, they can continue serving us well for years.

LET US GIVE THEM THE LOVE AND ATTENTION THEY DESERVE.

Remember, slight changes can lead to meaningful results. So, start making positive changes TODAY!

If you have acquired the necessary knowledge, why not begin your journey with the Renal Diet Cookbook?

LET US KNOW YOUR FEEDBACK AND EXPERIENCE WITH THIS RENAL DIET COOKBOOK.

Your feedback helps us improve and put it right in front of our readers.

WE APPRECIATE YOUR TIME, EFFORT, AND ENTHUSIASM!

PLEASE TAKE A FEW MINUTES TO SHARE YOUR EXPERIENCE
BY LEAVING A REVIEW ON AMAZON.

THANK YOU!

Author's Note

Hi there,

I wanted to take a moment to express my sincere gratitude for taking the time to read my book. As an author, there is no greater joy than knowing that my work has resonated with readers and provided some value to their lives. Your support means a great deal to me, and I am honored that you chose to read my book.

Thank you

Yours truly, **Emily**

Made in the USA
Las Vegas, NV
20 September 2023

77801868R00083